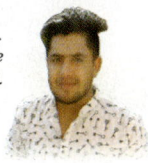

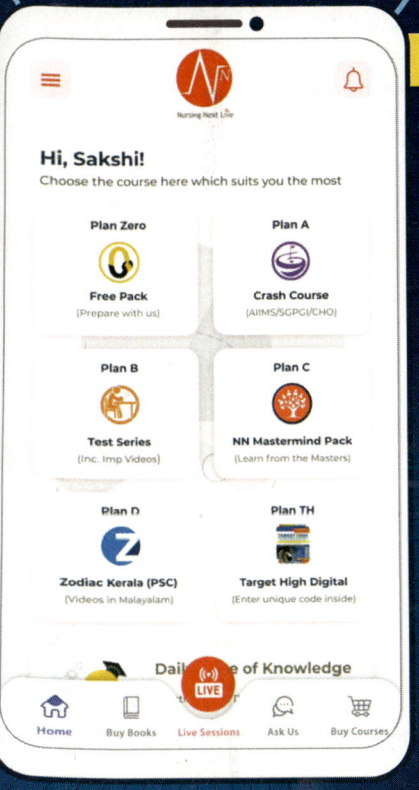
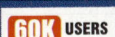 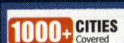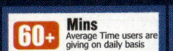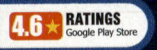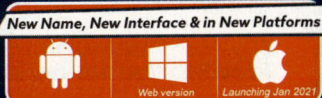

Nursing Next Live
Pack/Courses

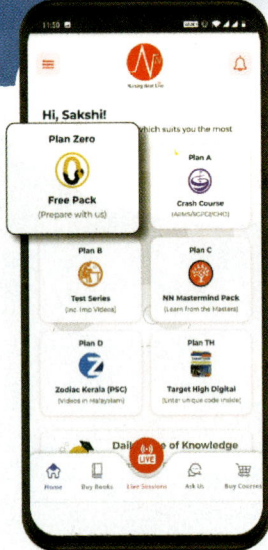

Plan ZERO : **FREE Pack** (Validity Unlimited)
What all you will get

- **2000+** MCQs with Rationale covering All Subjects, Important Topics
- **150+** E-Notes covering All Subjects, Selective important Topics
- **100+** Hours of Lectures covering All Subjects (Topic-wise/Imp Topics/Chanting/Exam Discussions)
- **100+** IBQS & VBQs of All Subjects
- **15** Most Recent/Previous Year Papers with Rationale (In Attempt/PDF)
- **5+** Grand Test & Bonus Test based on Real Time Exam Pattern
- Daily Dose of Word of the Day, Fact of the Day, Practice Pearls, Question of the Day
- Unsolved & Solved Question Papers of BSc 1st to 4th Year in a consolidated manner covering all Important Universities (Forthcoming)
- Monthly Scholarship Test with Special Prizes & Cash Back
- How to Prepare for Exams in the form of Study Planner/Videos
- Complete Access to Target High Extra Edge Section – which includes additional MCQs & Golden Points in Video Form

For more details and special offers log on to www.nursingnextlive.com

Plan A :
Crash Courses (Exam Centric)
What all you will get

Plan A1 – CHO Crash Course (Validity 60 Days)
- **32+** Subject-wise Tests & Grand Tests (including Bonus Tests & Previous Years Papers)
- **1500+** Questions with rationale
- **70+** E-notes for last minutes revision covering all the important topics as per the syllabus of CHO
- **30+** (Duration of 32+ Hours) Pre-recorded Videos given by top faculties in Hinglish covering every important topic from exam point of view

Plan A2 – AIIMS NORCET 2020 Crash Course (Validity 90 Days)
- **60+** Live Tests Subject-wise based on AIIMS Delhi pattern
- **1500+** Qs with Rationale including MCQs, IBQs, VBQs, Clinical skills, Priority setting, and case study
- **15+** Mock Test, Revision Test, and Grand Tests based on Real time pattern of AIIMS Delhi with Negative Marking and National Level Ranking
- All Subject-wise Tests & Grand Tests are with Detailed Rationales
- **140+** Last Minute Revision Notes based on Frequently asked Topics in previous Years
- **12+** Videos on Chanting Session by Top Educators/Subject Experts
- **35+** Multiple videos on special tricks for non-nursing subjects, tips on memory retention, strategies to attempt exams, etc.
- Success Guaranteed as we have had 150+ Selections (Rank 12 to 5k) in AIIMS NORCET 2020.

Plan A3 – Target Kerala PSC Crash Course (Validity 90 Days)
- **60+** Subject-wise/Grand Test with Rationale
- **320+** E-Notes in form of Subject-wise synopsis
- **50+** Hours of Videos in English (Important Topics Pre-loaded video + Chanting videos)
- In association with our Best-Selling Title - Target High Staff Nurse Entrance Exam

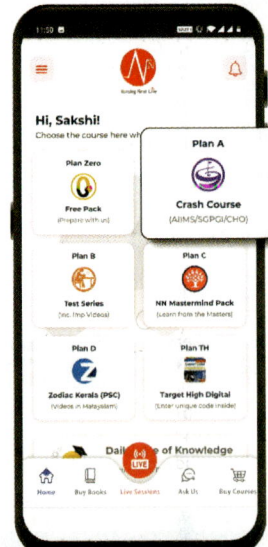

For more details and special offers log on to www.nursingnextlive.com

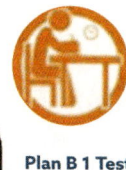

Plan B :
Test Series Ver 2.0
What all you will get

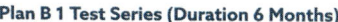

Plan B 1 Test Series (Duration 6 Months)

- **90+** Newly Created Subject-wise, Mini Test & Grand Test focusing all important National Exams AIIMS, PGIMER, JIPMER, DSSSB, RRB & ESIC (In 6 months)
- **6500+** Qs (MCQs, IBQs, VBQs) with Rationale & updated reference from standard textbooks. All the Tests are designed by the Subject Experts & Topper Students (In 6 months)
- **200+** Hours Recorded Video Lectures of Nursing/Non-Nursing Subjects by some of India's best nursing faculties/subject experts. Lectures are in English/Hindi language focusing on concept-based learning
- **5** Exam Discussion Videos of 2019 Exam papers (Duration 20 Hours)
- **150+** Hours of Recorded Video on Subject-wise Exam Discussion of previous years papers (2017-18) of all nursing exams delivered by subject experts
- **5** Skill Procedure videos demonstrating Nursing Skills in real-time
- **100+** Previous Year Exam Papers of all Nursing Exams from 2020-10 with Rationale (Attempt/View PDF Mode)
- **1500+** Flash cards on all the important topics of all the subjects for last minute revision (In 6 months)
- **800+** Image-based Questions with Rationale
- **150+** Video-based Qs with Rationale
- Includes complete content of current and upcoming crash courses

Plan B 2 Test Series (Duration 12 Months)

- **150+** Newly Created Subject-wise, Mini Test & Grand Test focusing all important National Exams AIIMS, PGIMER, JIPMER, DSSSB, RRB & ESIC (In 12 months)
- **10,000+** Qs (MCQs, IBQs, VBQs) with Rationale & updated reference from standard textbooks. All the Tests are designed by the Subject Experts & Topper Students (In 12 months)
- **200+** Hours Recorded Video Lectures of Nursing/Non-Nursing Subjects by some of India's best nursing faculties/subject experts. Lectures are in English/Hindi language focusing on concept-based learning
- **6** Exam Discussion Videos of 2020 Exam papers (Duration 25 Hours)
- **150+** Hours of Recorded Video on Subject-wise Exam Discussion of previous years papers (2017-18) of all nursing exams delivered by subject experts
- **5** Skill Procedure videos demonstrating Nursing Skills in real-time
- **120+** Previous Year Exam Papers of all Nursing Exams from 2020-10 with Rationale (Attempt/View PDF Mode) (In 12 Months)
- **1500+** Flash cards on all the important topics of all the subjects for last minute revision (In 12 Months)
- **1000+** Image-based Questions with Rationale
- **200+** Video-based Qs with Rationale
  Includes complete content of current and upcoming crash courses

For more details and special offers log on to www.nursingnextlive.com

Nursing Next Live
Pack/Courses

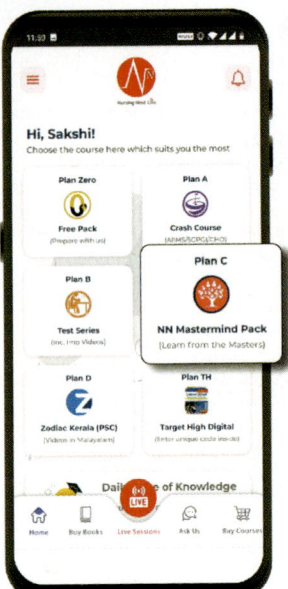

Plan C **plus:**
Nursing Next MASTERMIND Pack
(One in All, All in One)
Combined Pack - Includes Plan A & B (Validity 12 Months)

Special Features
- Nursing Next's **"NN Mastermind Pack"**, is a **One-Stop solution** for all your exam preparation needs for Staff Nurse Entrance Exams & Nursing Undergraduate Exams!
- It is our **One-in-All, All-in-One** pack for the nursing students of the Digital era!
- NN Mastermind Pack is exactly that 'learning tool' for all the nursing aspirants. It is carefully planned, and strategically designed, under the expertise of TOP Medical/Nursing Educators, just to make learning more authentic and easier for our students.
- Covering All Subjects, All Topics concepts from **Basics to Advance level** pattern with the help of Videos/Question Bank & Handwritten Notes
- The Masterminds (TOP EDUCATORS) of NN Live have focused on **ALL** the upcoming **Nursing Exams** by giving two convenient options of 'Individual pack', or 'Combined (NN Mastermind Pack)'
- **NN Mastermind** Pack is a "road to success" for those who are preparing either for the any and all **staff nurse entrance exams**.

What all you will get

Plan C plus (Inc. Plan A + Plan B)
- **1200+** hours of Video Lectures on All Subject/All Topics
- **11,000+** Questions with Rationale covering All Subject/All Topics
- **IBQs/VBQs** Video Discussions of All Subjects
- Monthly **Live Doubt** Sessions
- Rapid Revision Videos for **AIIMS NORCET 2021** (In July/August'21)
- **Handwritten Notes** of videos in PDF form will be integrated in the app by Feb '21
- Focusing on Quality study over quantity study, using the smart-study approach
- All the Content will be Live in **Four Phases in 4 Months** (Nov-Feb '21)
- All upcoming exams Important Topics & Exam/Discussions will be covered
- Complete 360 Approach for preparation
- Unlimited Time of Watch Time, FREE Download Video option, National Level Ranks, Bookmark the content, Pause & Resume
- **Best Guidance & Support at every stage**
- **+ Plan A of NN Live** (Complete access to Current & Upcoming Crash Courses)
- **+ Plan B of NN Live** (Complete access to Test Series Version 2.0)

Refer to Plan A & B for more details on the content included with Plan C plus

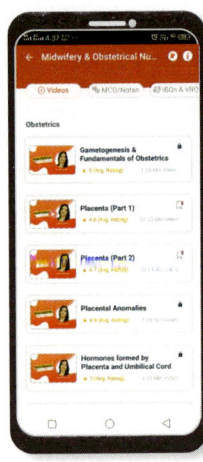
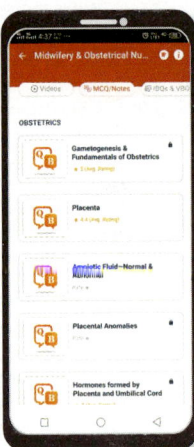

Nursing Next Mastermind Faculties

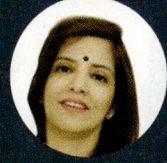

Dr. Sakshi Arora Hans
(Midwifery & Obstetrical Nursing)

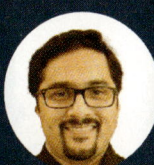

Dr. Rohan Khandelwal
(MSN–Surgery)

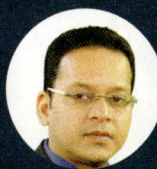

Dr. Ranjan Patel
(Pharmacology)

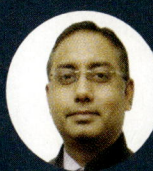

Dr. Mukhmohit Singh
(Community Health Nursing)

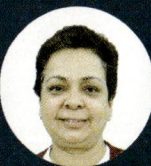

Dr. Shivika Sethi
(Microbiology)

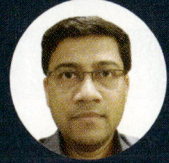

Dr. Ashish Kumar
(Physiology)

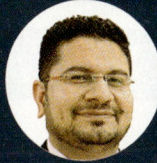

Dr. Aman Setiya
(MSN–Medicine)

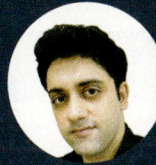

Dr. Anand Bhatia
(Pediatric Nursing)

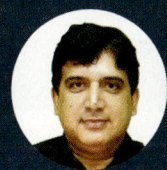

Dr. Dharmendra Singh
(Mental Health Nursing)

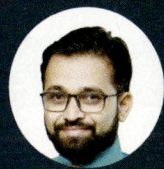

Dr. Shrikant Verma
(Anatomy)

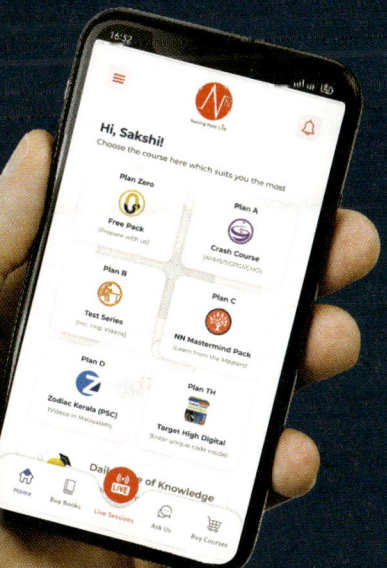

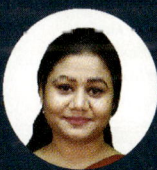

Dr. Karthikeyen Pethusamy
(Biochemistry & Nutrition)

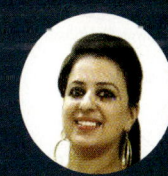

Ms. Sabina Ali
(FON, Nursing Research & Statistics)

Dr. Mrinalini Bakshi
(General English)

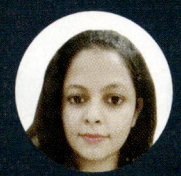

Ms. Priyanka Randhir
(Sociology & Computer)

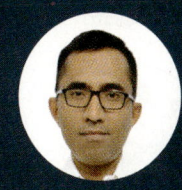

Mr. Nitish Dubey
(General Arithmetic)

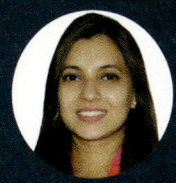

Ms. Saloni Sharma
(Aptitude & Reasoning)

TOP RANK HOLDERS

With over 150+ AIIMS NORCET 2020 Selections &

Say Hello to the
You can

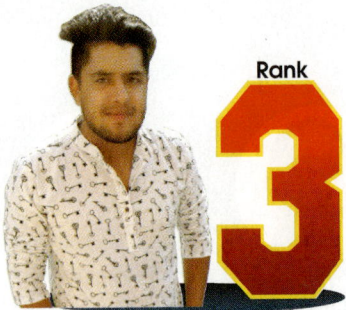

Rank

3

Rahul Dahiya
Roll No. 9016060

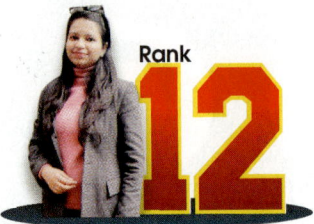

Rank

12

Nisha Singla
Roll No. 9101820

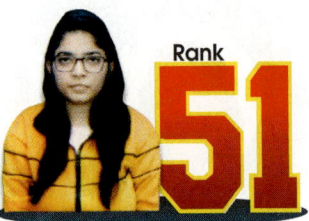

Rank

51

Komal Dhull
Roll No. 9024458

OUR ALL INDIA

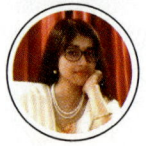

Saswati Bhommick
Rank - 141
Roll No. 9012620

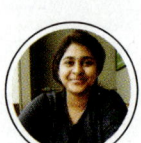

Sohini Mandal
Rank - 145
Roll No. 9042723

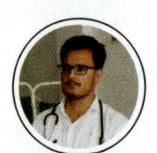

Divyanshu Khandelwal
Rank - 152
Roll No. 9011121

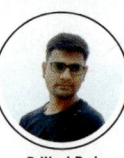

Prithvi Raj
Rank - 171
Roll No. 9030852

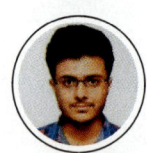

Ch. Prakash Kumar Nanjibhai
Rank - 244
Roll No. 9057267

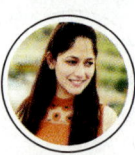

Arti
Rank - 245
Roll No. 9090452

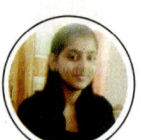

Annu Dahiya
Rank - 390
Roll No. 9005214

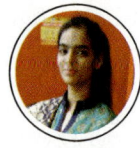

Shipra Choudhary
Rank - 417
Roll No. 9049237

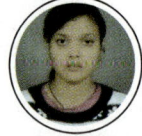

Pragya Maurya
Rank - 466
Roll No. 9033415

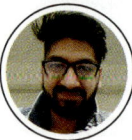

Mohan
Rank - 498
Roll No. 9090721

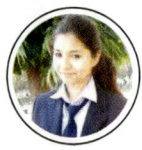

Rinki Negi
Rank - 519
Roll No. 9004223

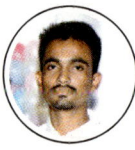

Om Leelawat
Rank - 523
Roll No. 9025575

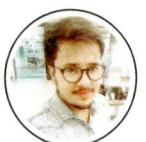

Mohammed Nadim
Rank - 803
Roll No. 9103198

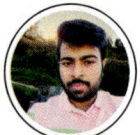

Abhas Singh
Rank - 822
Roll No. 9077010

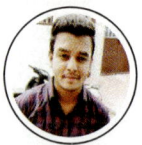

Kartavya Thaker
Rank - 827
Roll No. 9054007

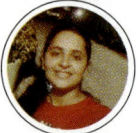

Sunita Goswami
Rank - 843
Roll No. 9060327

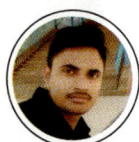

Dinesh Gehlot
Rank - 923
Roll No. 9043284

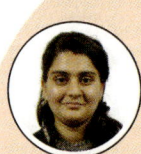

Surabhi Nandwana
Rank - 939
Roll No. 9091040

# of Nursing Next Live

NursingNextSquad!
be the Next . . .

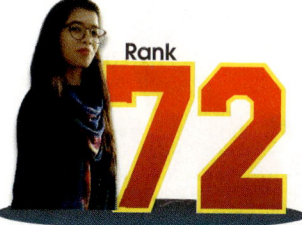

Rank 72

Shivani Bourai
Roll No. 9092877

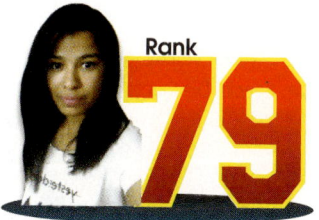

Rank 79

Nivedita Saini
Roll No. 9004587

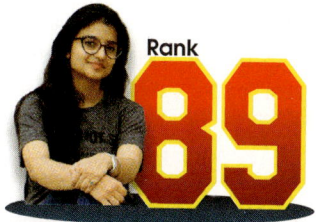

Rank 89

Rupali Garg
Roll No. 9054544

TOP RANKERS

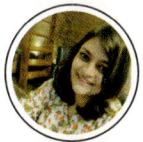

Mamta
Rank - 297
Roll No. 9063879

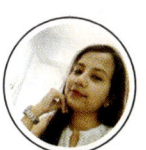

Neelam Rana
Rank - 328
Roll No. 9089800

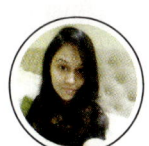

Gargi Baruah
Rank - 336
Roll No. 9019608

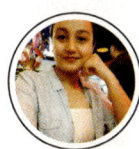

Parul Vats
Rank - 338
Roll No. 9027211

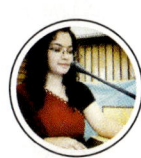

Anjull Chauhan
Rank - 367
Roll No. 9033536

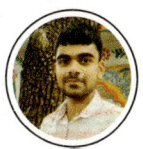

Vishal Gupta
Rank - 384
Roll No. 9023854

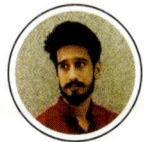

Sri Bhagwan
Rank - 540
Roll No. 9054478

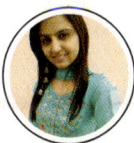

Jyoti Dhull
Rank - 560
Roll No. 9052005

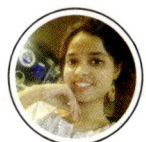

Sonia Mandal
Rank - 584
Roll No. 9007042

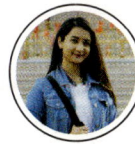

Pratibha Jhagta
Rank - 585
Roll No. 9093660

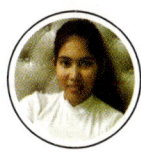

Arpita Pandey
Rank - 624
Roll No. 9087198

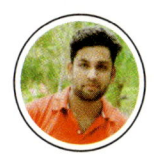

Vikram Prakash Kumhar
Rank - 745
Roll No. 9045800

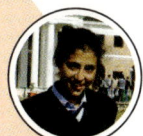

Ritu Tiwari
Rank - 947
Roll No. 9066617

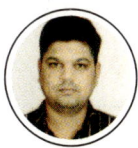

Himalay Choudhary
Rank - 1063
Roll No. 9094287

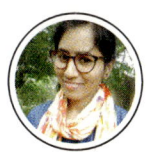

Swapnal Mallinath Sarne
Rank - 1197
Roll No. 9031619

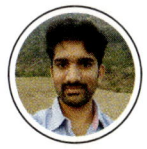

D.V. Ganapthi
Rank - 1317
Roll No. 9017393

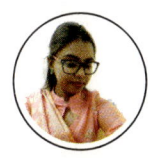

Varsha
Rank - 1330
Roll No. 9092296

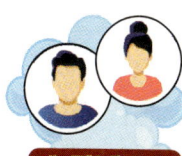

You Will Be The Next...

Why Follow Nursing Next Live On Social Media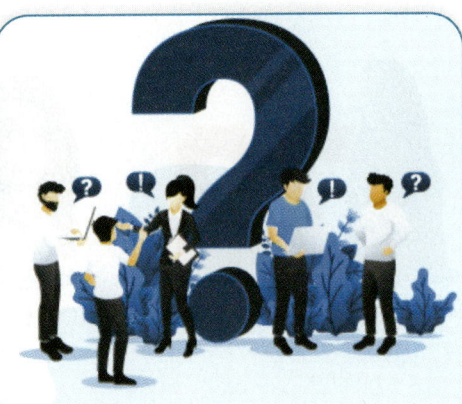

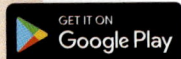 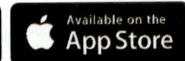

Procedure Manual for

Obstetric & Gynecological Nursing

Shweta Naik

MSc(N) Obstetrics & Gynecology

Assistant Lecturer
K J Somaiya College of Nursing
Sion, Mumbai

Hannah Roseline D

MSc(N) Obstetrics & Gynecology

Assistant Lecturer
K J Somaiya College of Nursing
Sion, Mumbai

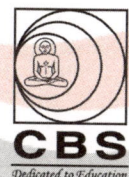

CBS
Dedicated to Education

CBS Publishers and Distributors Pvt Ltd

• New Delhi • Bengaluru • Chennai • Kochi • Kolkata • Mumbai
• Hyderabad • Nagpur • Patna • Pune • Vijayawada

Procedure Manual for

Obstetric & Gynecological Nursing

ISBN: 978-93-88178-60-0

Copyright © Publishers

First Edition: 2019

Published by **Satish Kumar Jain** and produced by **Varun Jain** for

CBS Publishers and Distributors Pvt Ltd

4819/XI Prahlad Street, 24 Ansari Road, Daryaganj, New Delhi 110 002, India.
Ph: 23289259, 23266861, 23266867   Website: www.cbspd.com
Fax: 011-23243014
e-mail: delhi@cbspd.com; cbspubs@airtelmail.in.
Corporate Office: 204 FIE, Industrial Area, Patparganj, Delhi 110 092
Ph: 4934 4934   Fax: 4934 4935
e-mail: bhupesharora@cbspd.com

Branches

- **Bengaluru:** Seema House 2975, 17th Cross, K.R. Road,
  Banasankari 2nd Stage, Bengaluru 560 070, Karnataka
  Ph: +91-80-26771678/79   Fax: +91-80-26771680
  e-mail: bangalore@cbspd.com

- **Chennai:** No. 7, Subbaraya Street, Shenoy Nagar, Chennai 600 030, Tamil Nadu
  Ph: +91-44-42032115   Fax: +91-44-42032115
  e-mail: chennai@cbspd.com

- **Kochi:** Ashana House, 39/1904, AM Thomas Road, Valanjambalam, Eranakulam 682 018, Kochi, Kerala
  Ph: +91-484-4059061-62-64-65   Fax: +91-484-4059065
  e-mail: kochi@cbspd.com

- **Kolkata:** No. 6/B, Ground Floor, Rameswar Shaw Road, Kolkata-700014 (West Bengal), India
  Ph: +91-33-2289-1126, 2289-1127
  e-mail: kolkata@cbspd.com

- **Mumbai:** 83-C, Dr E Moses Road, Worli, Mumbai-400018, Maharashtra
  Ph: +91-22-24902340/41   Fax: +91-22-24902342
  e-mail: mumbai@cbspd.com

Representatives

- Hyderabad   +91-9885175004
- Vijaywada   +91-74069-04007
- Nagpur   +91-9021734563
- Mangalore   +91-9741432102
- Patna   +91-9334159340

Printed At : Goyal Offset Printers

From Publisher's Desk

"Gaining knowledge is the first step to wisdom. Sharing it is the first step to humanity."

The above mentioned lines form the foundation stone of CBS publishers and Distributors Pvt Ltd, the flag bearer in medical publishing. Headquartered in New Delhi, the national capital of India, CBS was established in the year 1972 and it has expanded its roots to grow as a pioneer in the field of medical publishing in Asia. CBS is one of the largest and the fastest growing publishers of medical books in Southeast Asia. We are partners in the education of undergraduate and postgraduate students for we believe in nurturing the brains of medicos since the beginning of their careers in medicine. CBS joins the hands with the medical students as their first choice since the very moment they enter the college with BD Chaurasia's Human Anatomy and CC Chatterjee's Human Physiology. CBS is the proud owner of many bestselling titles like OP Ghai's Textbook of Pediatrics, Manipal's Surgery, KD Chatterjee's Textbook of Parasitology, and the list goes on. CBS has successfully partnered in sculpting the careers of millions of medicos across the world.

Since establishment of "CBS Nursing Knowledge Tree", we have published many successful titles in the field of nursing and we have proved ourselves in the nursing fraternity in providing Quality Education.

Vision and Mission of CBS Nursing Knowledge Tree

CBS Nursing Knowledge Tree is conceptualized with a vision of being the first of its kind to bring the best quality books for education of Nurses. Keeping in mind the changing trends in the Nursing Education, we at CBS have taken up a mission to bring student-friendly and syllabus-based books written by Subject Experts from PAN India without compromising on the Quality of content and presenting it in a Unique manner.

Foundation Stones of CBS Nursing Knowledge Tree

- **Strong editorial support by the leading subject experts and faculties in Nursing from PAN India.** Every manuscript/proposal that is received is critically reviewed by our Editorial Board at various levels to ensure the Quality of content. A book is published only after all the parameters in our process management are satisfied.

- **Special care taken to publish Plagiarism-free matter.** With the copyright laws being highly strict these days, we at CBS are paying extra attention at various stages of publishing a book to crosscheck and avoid any copyright infringement.

- **Books authored by Subject Experts and Senior Faculties all over India.** Every title owned by CBS Nursing Knowledge Tree is written by the senior-most faculties and subject masters from every nook and corner of the country to provide them a bigger platform to share their knowledge and experience amongst budding nursing fraternity.

- **All the books developed as per INC syllabus and needs of the students without compromising on the Quality of the content.** Often students complain that some books are either not covering the complete syllabus or have too much content as compared to the syllabus. In this series, extra care is being taken to develop books strictly as per INC syllabus in the most student-friendly manner.

- **All books being reviewed by Top-notch faculties and Subject Experts to maintain high standards of Quality.** Every title goes through tough grilling regarding the content and the overall presentation by various top subject experts as reviewers. This ensures that only the Quality content gets published.

- **Best International standard layouts for every book.** Every title in CBS Nursing Knowledge Tree is designed and formatted in the best layouts of international standards because we strongly believe that every book deserves to be treated the Best!
- **Additional and Unique features given with every title.** Every title is accompanied by one or the other additional feature to complement the learning of students like—*Workbook, DVD, Last Minute Revision Notes*. We have also included many features like *How to make Most out of this Book, Assess Yourself* that contains questions and MCQs and other special boxes according to the need of the content.

Let's Join Our Hands Together

We can only bring the change that we want to see in Nursing Education with the support and cooperation of leading faculties in all Nursing specialties. If you envision the same, we are happy to welcome you to our panel of contributors and reviewers and let's take up this mission together of creating a Change in Nursing Education.

We crave cooperation from all the students and faculties to provide their genuine feedback on the quality of the books and how we can improve upon the deficiencies in future on the following email id: cbsvpdesk@yahoo.com . Constructive criticism with concrete suggestions for improvement for all our books will be highly appreciated.

Expanding Horizons

We are also highly active in attending various National Level Conferences and Meets organized by various Nursing Societies. We are keenly working to expand our horizons of associations by participating in conferences organized by **SOCHNI, ISPN, NRSI, ICMR, SOMI,** etc. every year. CBS has always been a forerunner and a big supporter of all National level Nursing Conferences. *If you have any National and State level conference proposals, we are happy to be the part of these conferences.*

Being Social is Our Aspiration

In this era of Social Media, we are happy being social as well by bringing you our Facebook page 🆕 **facebook.com/cbsnursingtree** of "CBS Nursing Knowledge Tree" to expand our reach to the maximum people in Nursing. It is a platform purely dedicated to bring the important aspects and latest updates and developments in various domains and fields of Nursing. It will be our privilege if you could connect with us and share your knowledge and experiences as well on our Facebook page.

I would like to invite all the readers to come and join us on our facebook page and share some input, information and literature.

With this vision and above features we are happy to announce the release of Procedure Manual for Obstetric and Gynecological Nursing by Shweta Naik and Hannah Roseline D!

Bhupesh Arora

Vice President-Publishing and Marketing

(NURSING Division)

CBS Publishers and Distributors (Delhi) Pvt. Ltd.

Email: bhupesharora@cbspd.com

Mobile: (+91) 9555590180

Preface

Till now there are many nursing procedure manuals available, but as such there is no separate manual for obstetric and gynecological nursing where student can clarify their doubts in this field. There is an increasing need of the procedure manual which is especially for obstetric and gynecological nursing.

This felt need motivated us to write a comprehensive "Procedure Manual of Obstetric and Gynecological Nursing" which is precised and put emphasis on common procedures, instruments and health advice. The book has been organized in such a way that it will help the students to improve their knowledge and develop their skills in midwifery practice.

This procedure manual is written in simple, clear, concise language with explanations and diagrams. This book would be extremely useful for the students, teachers and nurses in the clinical side.

Shweta Naik

Hannah Roseline D

Acknowledgments

Firstly we thank the almighty for enabling us to complete this Procedure Manual for Obstetric and Gynecological Nursing. We take this great opportunity to thank those who have contributed in writing this manual.

It was our long awaited dream to write a "Procedure Manual for Obstetric and Gynecological Nursing" procedures and this was made success only due to Mrs Avani Oke, Principal of KJ Somaiya School and College of Nursing, whose constant encouragement, constructive inputs and untiring support gave us inspiration and motivation to write and publish this procedure manual.

We would like to acknowledge Dr Geeta Niyogi, Dr Rajeshwari for their quality inputs and coordinating corrections in the procedure manual. We are thankful to our colleagues in our institution for their aspiration and support.

Also we would like to mention the contributions of 4th year Basic BSc Nursing batch 2017–2018 in preparation of the book.

Thanks to our family members, as they deserve much more credits for our accomplishments.

We appreciate support of **Mr Satish Kumar Jain** (*Chairman*) and **Mr Varun Jain** (*Managing Director*), M/s CBS Publishers and Distributors Pvt Ltd. for their whole-hearted support in publication of this book. No amount of words can describe role, efforts, inputs and initiatives undertaken by **Mr Bhupesh Arora**, (*Vice President-Publishing and Marketing, PGMEE and Nursing Division*), for his endeavor toward the development of the book.

We thank Dr Mrinalini Bakshi (Sr Content Developer and Editor) for her editorial support and Ms Nitasha Arora (Project Manager), Ms Neetu Jindal (Asst. Production Manager), Mr Nitish K Dubey (Senior Editor) and all the production team members Mr Ashutosh Pathak, Mr Chaman Lal, Mr Phool Kumar, Mr Bunty Kashyap, Mr Prakash Gaur, Ms Tahira Praveen, Ms Babita Verma, Mr Raju Sharma, Vikram Chaudhary, Manoj Chaudhary, Manoj Malakar and Chander for devoting laborious hours in designing and typesetting of this book. We convey thanks to all those who are associated with this book.

Contents

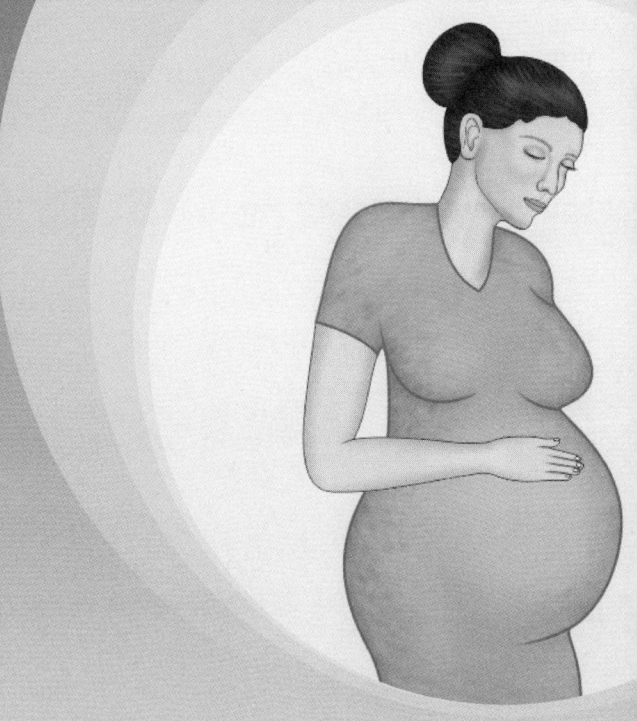

ANTENATAL PROCEDURES

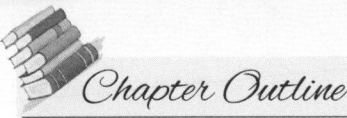

Chapter Outline

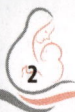

ANTENATAL ASSESSMENT

Purposes

- To assess pregnancy-related changes in mother
- To notify any deviation from normal changes
- To identify high-risk pregnancy case.

Equipments Needed

A clean tray containing the following articles (**Figs 1 and 2**):

- Thermometer
- Stethoscope
- Sphygmomanometer
- Scale for height measurement
- Weighing machine
- Measuring tape
- Knee hammer
- Gloves
- Bowl containing spirit/Savlon swabs
- Paper bag
- Kidney tray
- Torch

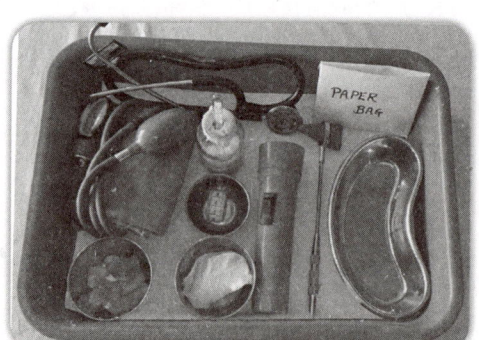

Fig. 1: A tray containing articles for antenatal assessment

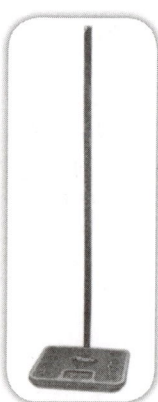

Fig. 2: Height and weight assessment

Procedure

Steps of procedure	Rationale
• Perform hand washing	• To prevent cross infection
• Provide privacy to patient	• To ensure safe and secure feel for patient
• Check vital signs of patient (temperature, pulse, respirations and blood pressure) (**Fig. 3**)	• To obtain patient's baseline data
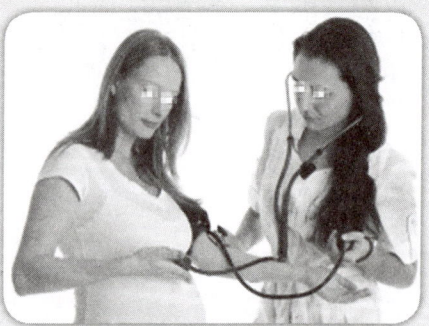 **Fig. 3:** Assessing vital parameters	
• Measure height, weight and BMI of patient	• Height to assess for short stature, weight for assessing weight gain during pregnancy

Contd...

Steps of procedure	Rationale

• Perform head-to-toe physical assessment and look for following features:
 	
  ▪ **General appearance:** Sick/Active/Anemic/Pallor
  ▪ **Systemic Examination**
  ▪ **Respiratory system (RS):**_____
  _____
  ▪ **Cardiovascular system (CVS):** _____
  _____
  ▪ **Gastrointestinal system (GI):** _____
  _____
 	
  ▪ **Body build:** Moderate/Thin/Obese
  ▪ **Head:** Normal/Dandruff/Pediculosis/Flakes/ Dryness/Itching
  ▪ **Hair texture:** Normal/Brittle/Easily pluckable
  ▪ **Face:** Pregnancy mask/puffiness/facial edema
  ▪ **Eyes**
    ○ **Pupil:** Normal/Dilated/Constricted
    ○ **Conjunctiva:** Red/Pale/Pink
    ○ **Sclera:** White/Icterus
  ▪ **Ears:** Normal/Wax impaction/Abnormal articular development
  ▪ **Nose:** Normal/Nasal septal Deviation/Nasal polyp/ Rhinitis
  ▪ **Lips:** Normal/Cheilosis/Dry/Pale
  ▪ **Tongue:** Fissures/Glossitis/Coated/Normal
  ▪ **Neck:** Thyroid enlargement
      Jugular veins distension
      Cervical lymphadenopathy
  ▪ **Breasts:** Symmetry/Distended veins/Areola/ Nipple type/Montogmery's tubercle/Consistency/ Secretion/Any palpable mass
  ▪ **Abdomen:**
    ○ **Inspection:** Abdominal size/Shape/Contour/ Linea nigra/ Striae gravidarum/Straie albicans/ Fetal movements/Distended veins/Umbilicus abnormalities/previous scar/Edema
    ○ **Palpation:** Measure fundal height and abdominal girth/Fundal grip/Left and right lateral grips/ Pelvic grip/Pawlic grip
    ○ **Auscultation:** Locate and measure fetal heart sound (FHS)
  ▪ **Back:** Lordosis/Backache
  ▪ **Hands:** Symmetry/Movements/Any deviation
  ▪ **Legs:** Symmetry/Movements/Varicosity/Edema/ Any deviation
  ▪ **Perineum:** Edema/Varicose veins/Vaginal discharge/Previous Scar
	• To assess physical and physiological changes during pregnancy.

• Replace all articles. • Do recording and reporting.	• As per basic principle of good workmanship. • To ensure SMART documentation.

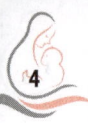

Points to Remember

- Mother should be comfortable and relax
- Ensure adequate privacy for mother
- Have a female attendant compulsory, if examined by male candidate
- Always compare with previous assessment findings, e.g. weight.

ANTENATAL PALPATION

Purposes

- To perform abdominal palpation
- To locate fetal heart sound (FHS)
- To notify any deviation from normal changes

Equipments Needed

A clean tray containing following articles (**Fig. 4**):

- Stethoscope/Fetoscope
- Measuring tape
- Gloves (for infectious patient)
- Bowl containing spirit swabs
- Paper bag
- Kidney tray

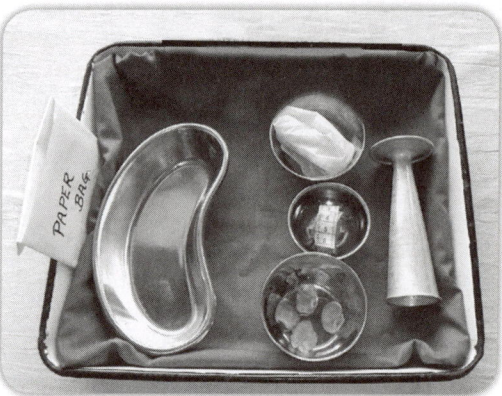

Fig. 4: A tray containing articles for antenatal palpation

Procedure

Steps of procedure	Rationale
• Ask patient to evacuate bladder and to relax perineal muscles	• Bladder evacuation to optimize patient's comfort whereas relaxing perineal muscles will reduce procedural pain and ease of procedure
• Give dorsal position to patient and tell her flexed legs a bit	• To allow easy examination of pelvic area
• Perform hand washing	• To prevent cross infection
• Provide privacy to patient	• To ensure safe and secure feel for patient
• Warm hands before touching abdomen and do not remove hands from abdomen till you complete the palpation	• To prevent fetal stimulation by cold hand
• Perform palpation with finger pads and not with finger tips (**Fig. 5**).	• To ensure accurate findings

Contd...

Steps of procedure	Rationale
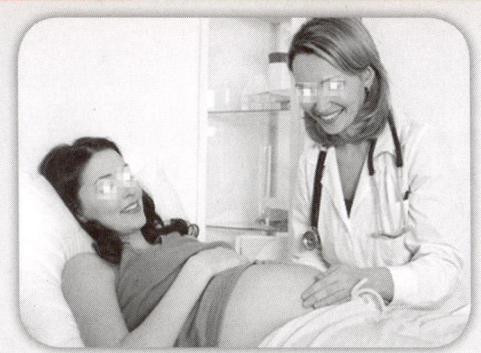 **Fig. 5:** Abdominal palpation	
• Check abdominal girth (AG) at umbilicus level and also check for symphysofundal height (SFH) in centimeters (**Fig. 6**)	• To assess increase in AG and SFH as per gestational age of patient
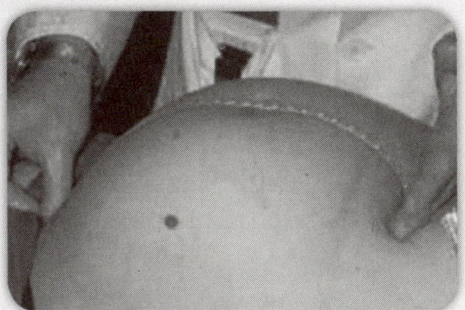 **Fig. 6:** Measuring symphysofundal height	

• Perform abdominal palpation
  ■ **Abdomen:**
    ○ **Inspection:** Abdominal size/Shape/Contour/ Linea nigra/Striae gravidarum/Straie albicans/ Fetal movements/Distended veins/Previous scar/Edema (**Fig. 7**)
	• To examine maternal changes during pregnancy and for assessing Fetus in utero

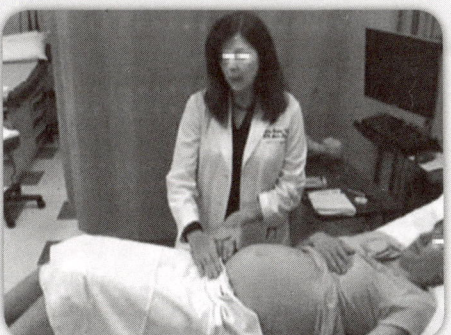 **Fig. 7:** Abdominal inspection	

Contd...

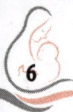

Steps of procedure	Rationale
○ **Palpation:** Measures fundal height and abdominal girth/Fundal grip/Left and right lateral grips/Pelvic grip/Pawlic grip. Palpate with finger pads (**Figs 8A to D**)	

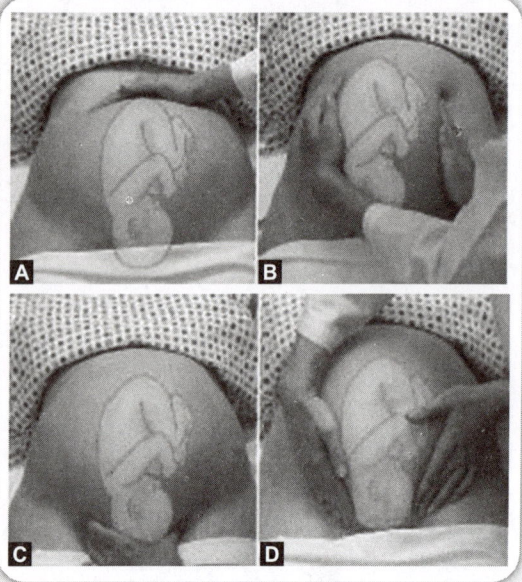

Figs 8A to D: Illustration showing abdominal palpation

○ **Auscultation:** Locate and count fetal heart sound (FHS) per minute (**Fig. 9**)

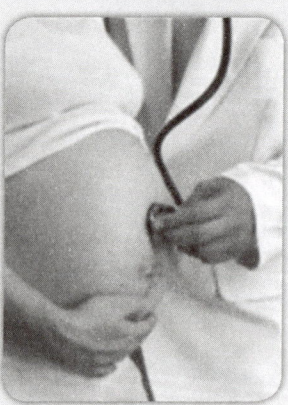

Fig. 9: Auscultation

- **Interpretation of results:** In left occiput anterior (LOA) position
  - **Fundal Grip:** Soft, round, ballotable part indicating fetal buttock
  - **Left lateral grip:** Curved, continuous, resistance felt part indicating fetal back

- To assess fetal wellbeing in utero and to detect any abnormal lie/position/presentation

Contd...

Steps of procedure	Rationale
▪ **Right lateral grip:** Small, irregular, knob like structures indicating fetal limbs ▪ **Pelvic grip:** Hard, round, ballotable/non-ballotable part indicating fetal head ▪ **Lie:** Longitudinal ▪ **Presentation:** Cephalic ▪ **Position:** LOA ▪ **Attitude:** Flexion ▪ **FHS:** _____/min	
• Replace all articles	• As per basic principle of good workmanship
• Do recording and reporting	• To ensure SMART documentation

Points to Remember

- Mother should be comfortable and relax
- Ensure adequate privacy for mother
- Have a female attendant compulsory, if examined by male candidate
- Bladder should be evacuated prior the procedure
- Mother should relax and not to contract abdominal muscles
- Always compare with previous assessment findings, e.g. AG, SFH, etc..

ANTENATAL BREAST EXAMINATION

Purposes

- To examine pregnancy-related breast changes.
- To notify any deviation from normal changes.

Equipments Needed

A clean tray containing the following articles (**Fig. 10**):

- Bowl containing warm water
- Bowl containing 4 Gamgy Pads
- Gauge piece - 2
- Trukese Napkin-1
- Pair Gloves -1
- Kidney tray
- Paper bag

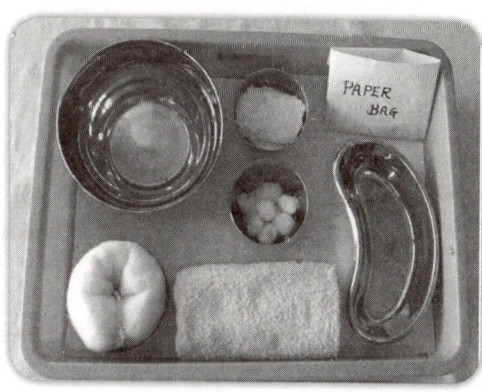

Fig. 10: A tray containing article for breast care

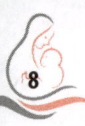
Procedure

Steps of procedure	Rationale
• Give supine/sitting position to patient	• To facilitate ease during procedure
• Perform hand washing	• To prevent cross infection
• Provide privacy to patient	• To ensure safe and secure feel for patient
• Perform breast inspection and palpation examination and look for: **Breasts:** Symmetry/distended veins/areola/nipple type/Montgomery's tubercle/consistency/secretion/any palpable mass (**Fig. 11**) 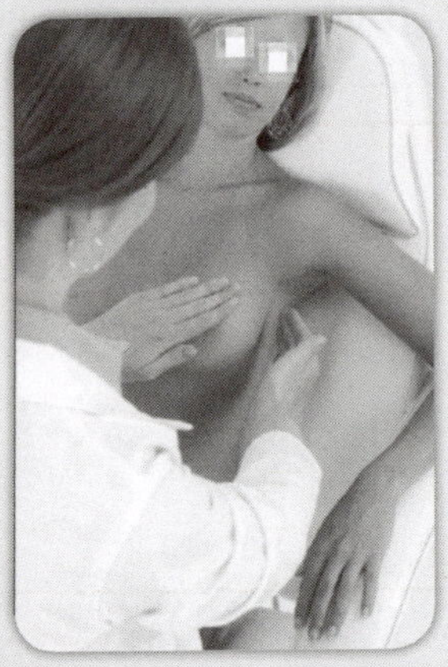	• To notify any deviation from normal

Fig. 11: Assessment of breasts

• Perform breast and axilla palpation with finger pads to detect any mass or lump (**Figs 12A to C**)	• To palpate for enlarge axillary lymph nodes

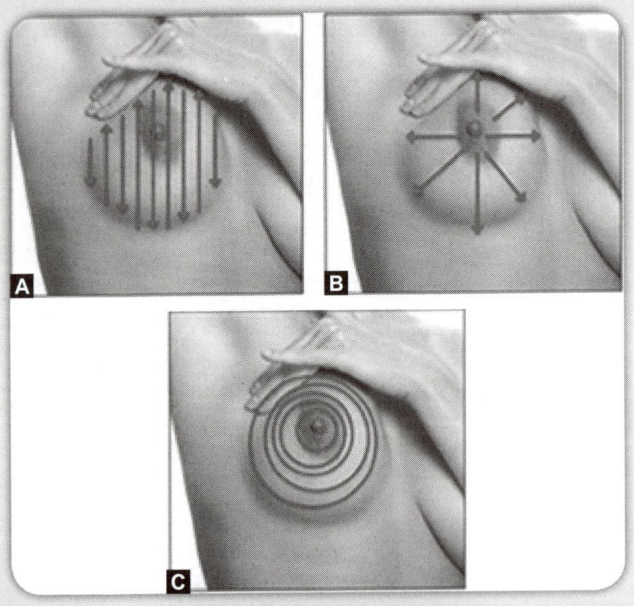

Figs 12A to C: Methods of breast assessment: A. Vertical method; B. Radial method; C. Spiral method

Contd...

Steps of procedure	Rationale
• Replace all articles	• As per basic principle of good workmanship
• Do recording and reporting	• To ensure SMART documentation

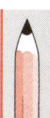

Points to Remember

- Mother should be comfortable and relax
- Ensure adequate privacy for mother
- Have a female attendant compulsory, if examined by male candidate.

URINE PREGNANCY TEST

Purpose

To confirm pregnancy

Equipments Needed

A clean tray containing following the articles (**Fig. 13**):

- Urine pregnancy test (UPT) kit
- Dropper
- Sample bottle containing urine
- Gloves
- Paper bag
- Kidney tray

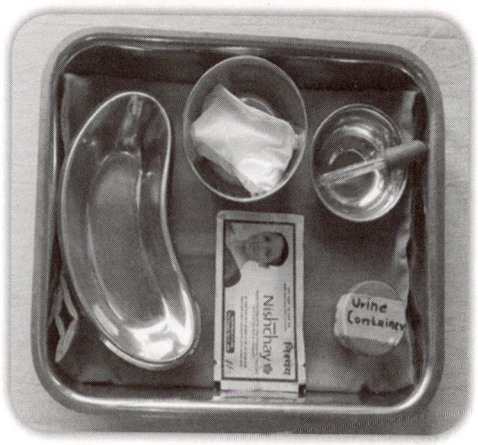

Fig. 13: A tray for urinary pregnancy test

Procedure

Steps of procedure	Rationale
• Perform hand washing and wear gloves	• To prevent cross infection
• Put 2–3 drops of urine in sample window of kit	• To perform urine pregnancy test
• Keep it for 5 minutes and then see for control and test lines (**Fig. 14**)	• To obtain accurate result

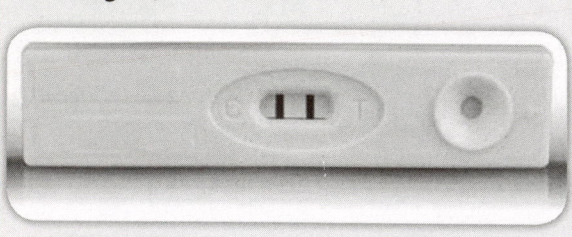

Fig. 14: Urine pregnancy test (UPT) positive reading

Contd...

Steps of procedure	Rationale
• If both are pigmented test is positive and if only control line is pigmented test is negative (**Fig. 15**)	• To interpret accurate finding.
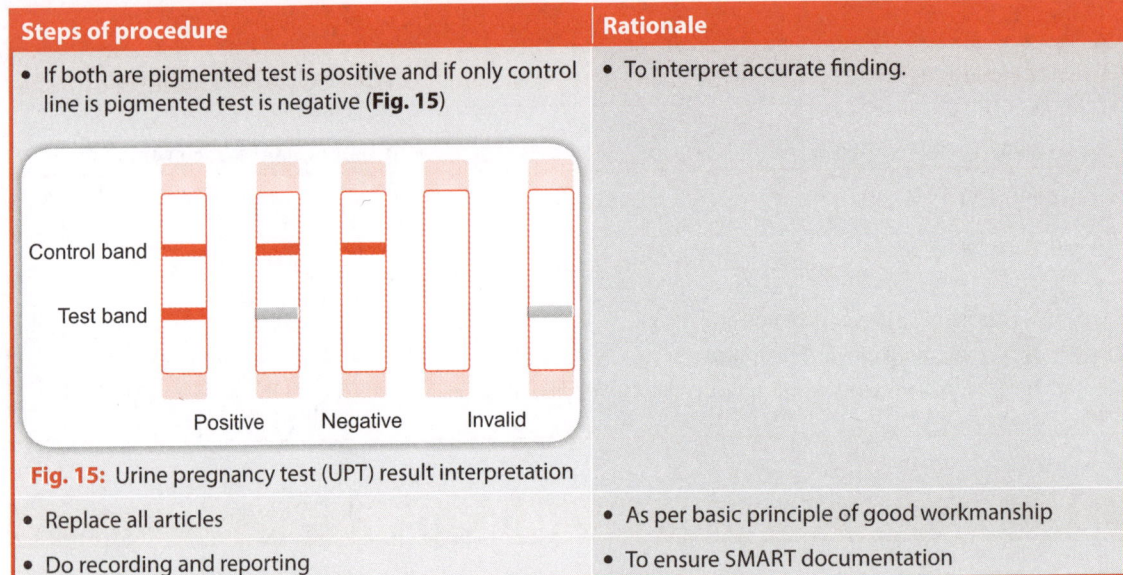 **Fig. 15:** Urine pregnancy test (UPT) result interpretation	
• Replace all articles	• As per basic principle of good workmanship
• Do recording and reporting	• To ensure SMART documentation

Points to Remember

- Most preferably collect morning urine sample
- Take midstream urine in clean container
- Read manufactures' order for the procedure
- If test is weakly positive, retest to be done a weak after
- Uterine pregnancy to be confirmed with ultrasonography.

URINE ALBUMIN TEST

Dipstick Method

Purpose

To assess urine albumin level.

Equipments Needed

A clean tray containing the following articles (**Fig. 16**):

- Dipsticks
- Sample bottle containing urine
- Gloves
- Paper bag
- Kidney tray

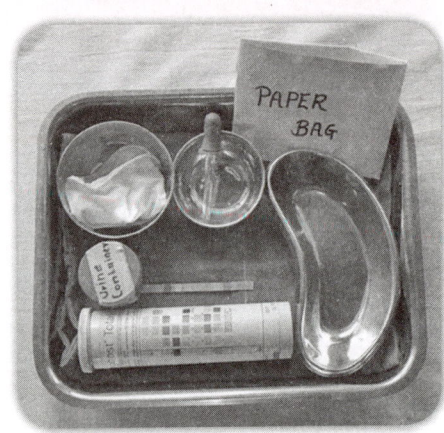

Fig. 16: A tray containing articles for urine albumin test

Procedure

Steps of procedure	Rationale
• Perform hand washing	• To prevent cross infection
• Wear gloves	• To prevent cross infection
• Dip dipstick in urine sample	• To perform urine albumin test
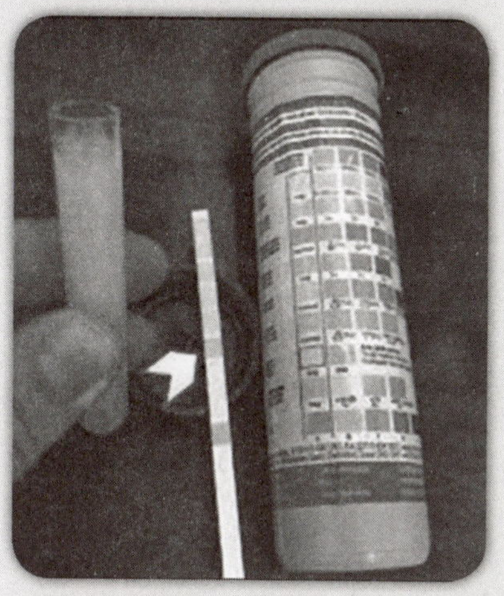 • Read result for urine albumin at given time as per manufacturers order (**Fig. 17**)	• To interpret accurate finding

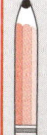

Fig. 17: Result interpretation

• Replace all articles	• As per basic principle of good workmanship
• Do recording and reporting	• To ensure SMART documentation

Points to Remember

- Most preferably collect morning urine sample
- Take midstream urine in clean container
- Read manufactures' order for the procedure
- Interpret with proper color match on manufacture's bottle
- Compare with previous findings.

Cold Test

Purpose

To assess urine albumin level

Equipments Needed

A clean tray containing the following articles:

- Bottle containing sulfosalicylic acid (SSA) with dropper
- Clear glass sample bottle/test tube containing urine

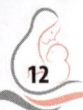
- Gloves
- Paper bag
- Kidney tray

Procedure

Steps of procedure	Rationale
• Perform hand washing	• To prevent cross infection
• Wear gloves	• To prevent cross infection
• In test tube/specimen bottle containing urine squirt an equal amount of 3% SSA into the tube directly on top of the urine. (½ – 1 mL each is required)	• To perform urine albumin test
• Shake tube gently with a quick flick and read for turbidity immediately (**Fig. 18**) NEG Trace 1+ 2+ 3+ 4+ **Fig. 18:** Result interpretation	• To interpret accurate finding
• Replace all articles	• As per basic principle of good workmanship
• Do recording and reporting	• To ensure SMART documentation

Points to Remember

- Most preferably collect morning urine sample
- Take midstream urine in clean container
- Interpret results by assessing degree of turbidity
- Compare with previous findings.

URINE SUGAR TEST

Purpose

To assess urine sugar level

Equipments Needed

A clean tray containing the following articles (**Fig. 19**):

- Dipsticks
- Sample bottle containing urine
- Gloves
- Paper bag
- Kidney tray

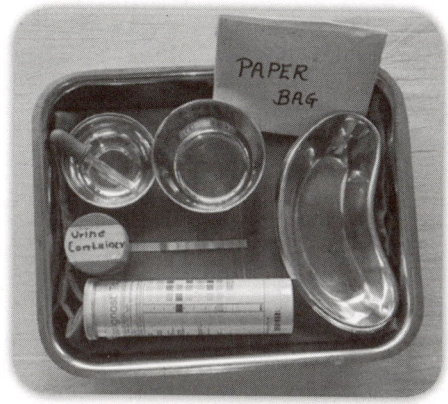

Fig. 19: A tray containing articles for urine sugar test

Procedure

Steps of procedure	Rationale
• Perform hand washing	• To prevent cross infection
• Wear gloves	• To prevent cross infection
• Dip dipstick in urine sample	• To perform urine sugar test
• Read result for urine sugar at given time as per manufacturers order	• To interpret accurate finding
• Replace all articles (**Fig. 20**)	• As per basic principle of good workmanship
Fig. 20: Result interpretation	
• Do recording and reporting	• To ensure SMART documentation

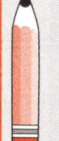 *Points to Remember*

- Most preferably collect morning urine sample
- Take midstream urine in clean container
- Read manufactures' order for the procedure
- Interpret with proper color match on manufacture's bottle
- Compare with previous findings.

NOTE

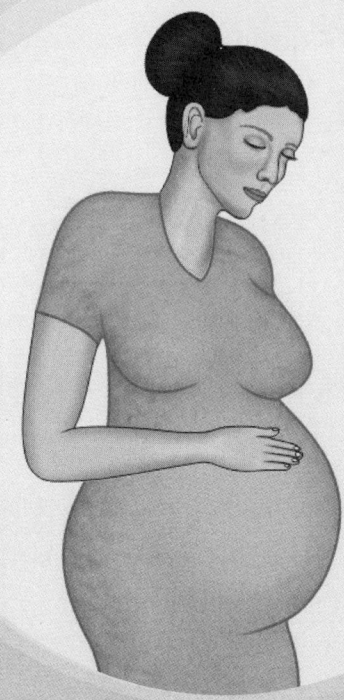

INTRANATAL PROCEDURES

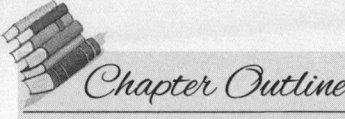

Chapter Outline

PERVAGINAL EXAMINATION

Purposes

- To diagnose labor
- To rule out cephalopelvic disproportion (CPD)
- To detect cervical dilatation and effacement
- To assess presence or absence of bag of membrane
- To rupture bag of membrane
- To determine color of amniotic fluid
- To confirm presenting part
- To assess station of part of presentation
- To exclude abnormal presentation like shoulder, cord, etc.

Equipments Needed

A sterile tray containing the following articles (**Fig. 1**):

- Gloves
- Bowl containing Savlon swabs
- Bowl containing normal saline swabs.
- A bowl containing Gauze piece.
- Kocher's forceps (to rupture bag of membrane)
- Kidney tray

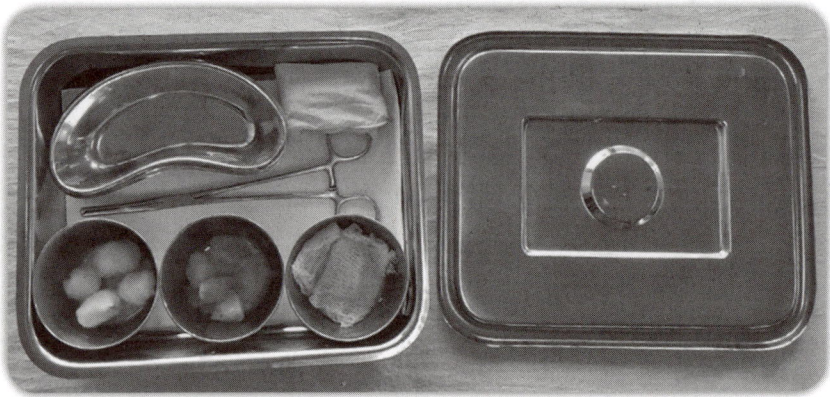

Fig. 1: A tray containing articles for pervaginal examination

Procedure

Steps of procedure	Rationale
• Provide privacy to patient	• To ensure safe and secure feel for patient
• Give dorsal position with flexed knees to patient	• To allow easy examination of pelvic area
• Perform hand washing	• To prevent cross infection
• Wear gloves aseptically	• To prevent cross infection

Contd...

Steps of procedure	Rationale
• Paint perineum with left hand from upward to downward and from inner to outer direction with Savlon and normal saline respectively	• Painting perineum ensures sterility of examination area and prevents ascending infection, whereas use of left hand for painting maintains sterility of dominant working hand (right hand)
• Hold index and middle finger of right hand close to each other and insert it in introitus while separating labia with gauze by other hand	• To ensure ease of procedure, maintains sterility of examination fingers and to reduce procedural pain
• After inserting two fingers, separate it and assess for findings **(Figs 2 and 3)**	• To assess accurate findings

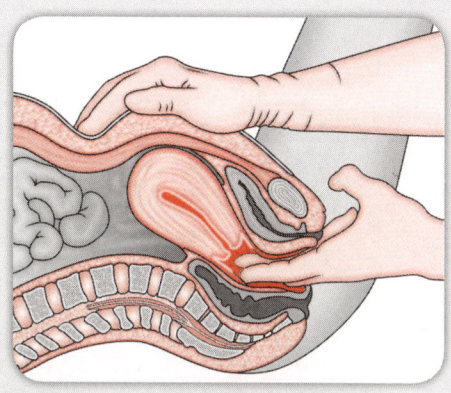

Fig. 2: Pervaginal examination

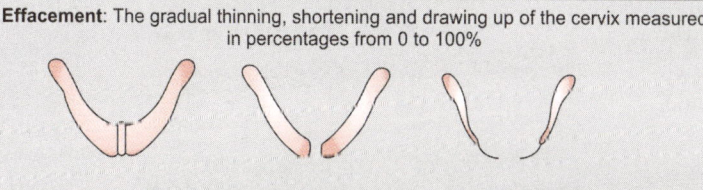

Effacement: The gradual thinning, shortening and drawing up of the cervix measured in percentages from 0 to 100%

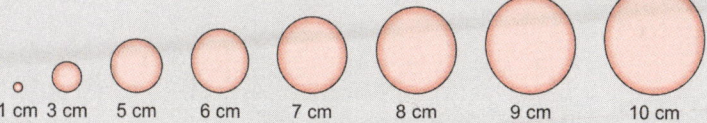

Dilation: The gradual opening of the cervix measured in centimeters from 0 to 10 cms

1 cm 3 cm 5 cm 6 cm 7 cm 8 cm 9 cm 10 cm

Fig. 3: Assessing cervical dilatation and effacement

• While removing fingers after completion of PV examination, bring finger together and remove it.	• To ensure ease of procedure and prevent injury
• Replace all articles	• As per basic principle of good workmanship
• Do recording and reporting	• To ensure SMART documentation

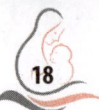

MAINTENANCE OF PARTOGRAPH

Purposes

- To assess progress of labor
- To provide details of necessary information, i.e. Parameters of fetomaternal wellbeing maternal welbeing and labor progress
- To predict deviation from normal duration of labor
- To take necessary action in case of prolonged labor (instrumental/operative delivery).

Equipments Needed (Fig. 4)

- Vital signs assessment tray
- Pervaginal examination tray (**Fig. 5**)
- Medication tray/pie dish (if required)
- Doppler with jelly and cotton swabs
- Partograph
- Three color pens, pencil and scale

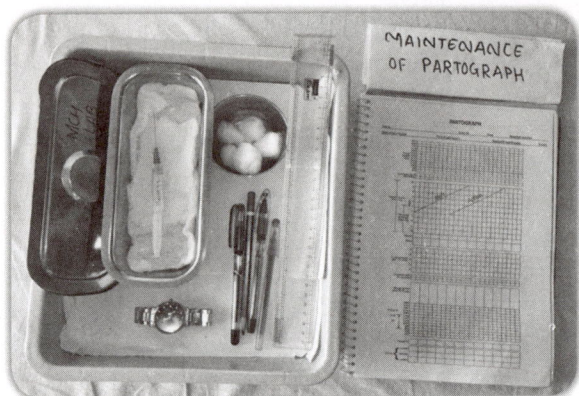

Fig. 4: A tray containing articles for maintenance of partograph

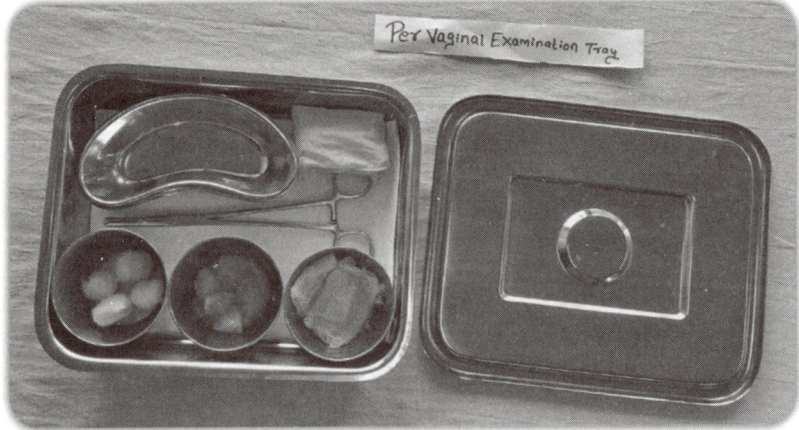

Fig. 5: A tray containing articles for pervaginal examination

Procedure

Steps of procedure	Rationale
• Throughout the labor achieve patient's optimal comfort	• To ensure patient's optimal cooperation
• Provide privacy to patient	• To ensure safe and secure feel for patient
• Perform hand washing before and after each procedure	• To prevent cross infection
• Start plotting Partograph once patient is in active phase of labor, i.e. cervical dilatation 4 cm and more. (WHO guidelines). Also maintain time and duration of recording	• To ensure accurate timely recording and prevent any error
• Fill demographic data of mother	• To ensure right documentation for right patient

• Assess following findings
 ▪ **Fetal heart sound (FHS):**
  ○ Record FHS with **red** cross 1 hourly in transient phase, every 30 minutes in active phase and every 15 minutes in second stage of labor
 ▪ **Amniotic fluid (blue ink):**
  ○ Intact membrane **'I'**
  ○ Clear liquor **'C'**
  ○ Meconium stained liquor **'M'**
  ○ Blood stained liquor **'B'**
 ▪ **Molding (blue ink):**
  ○ Parietal bones touching+
  ○ Parietal bones overlapping ++
  ○ Parietal bones overlapping severely +++
 ▪ **Cervical dilatation and descent of fetal head (Pencil)**
  ○ Perform pervaginal examination and plot cervical dilatation and descent against time
  ○ In active phase of labor 4 hourly PV examination is permitted **(Fig. 6)**
 ▪ **Contractions per 10 minutes (Pencil)**
  ○ Keep palm of hand on fundus of uterus and assess for duration of uterine contractions
  ○ Also count number of contractions in 10 minutes and plot it
  ○ Less than 20 sec **Mild contractions** [::::::]
  ○ 20–40 sec **moderate contractions** [//////]
  ○ More than 40 sec **severe contractions** [▮]
 ▪ **Oxytocin (blue ink)**
  ○ Maintain chart of oxytocin unit per litre and drops per minute against time
 ▪ **Drugs/IV medications (red ink)**
  ○ Record drugs or IV fluids given during labor
	• To ensure maternal-fetal wellbeing and record progress of labor as well to detect the high-risk cases requiring instrumental or operative interferences

Contd...

Steps of procedure	Rationale
▪ **Maternal vital signs (pulse red ink rest in blue)** ○ Assess maternal vital signs (Temperature, Pulse and BP) 1–2 hourly and record it ▪ **Urine (blue ink)** ○ Measure urine volume (In high risk patients) ○ Test for urine acetone/protein, if required	
• **Points to be remember** ▪ Cervical dilatation line graph should always be normal (i.e. **Above alert line**) ▪ If it is between **alert** and **action line** most probably delivery aided by drugs and instrumentation ▪ If it crosses action line then mother shifted for operative delivery	• To detect high-risk cases requiring instrumental or operative interferences
• After delivery write a brief delivery note on right side of partograph	• To ensure completeness of recording
• Replace all articles	• As per basic principle of good workmanship
• Do recording and reporting	• To ensure SMART documentation

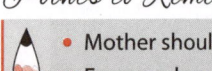

Points to Remember

- Mother should be comfortable and relaxed
- Ensure adequate privacy for mother
- Have a female attendant compulsory, if examined by male candidate
- Give adequate explanation and positive reinforcement during procedure as it may be painful
- Inform progress of findings to patient
- Report any deviation from normal progress to doctor immediately.
- Always compare with previous assessment findings.

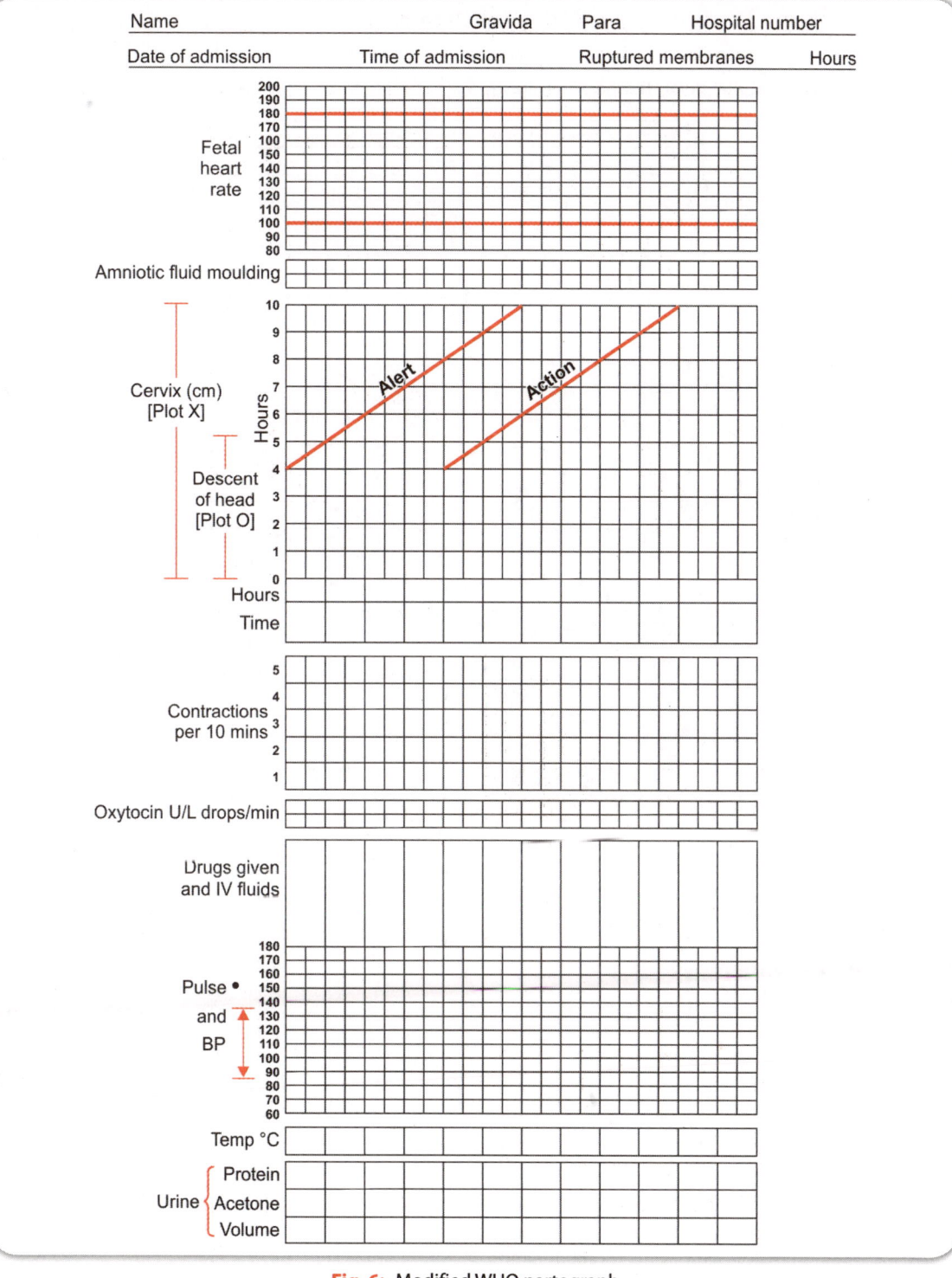

Fig. 6: Modified WHO partograph

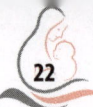

Partograph Recording

Name ABC Gravida 5 Para 2 Hospital number 4570

Date of admission 20/9/17 Time of admission 02:27 pm Ruptured membranes 02:27 pm Hours

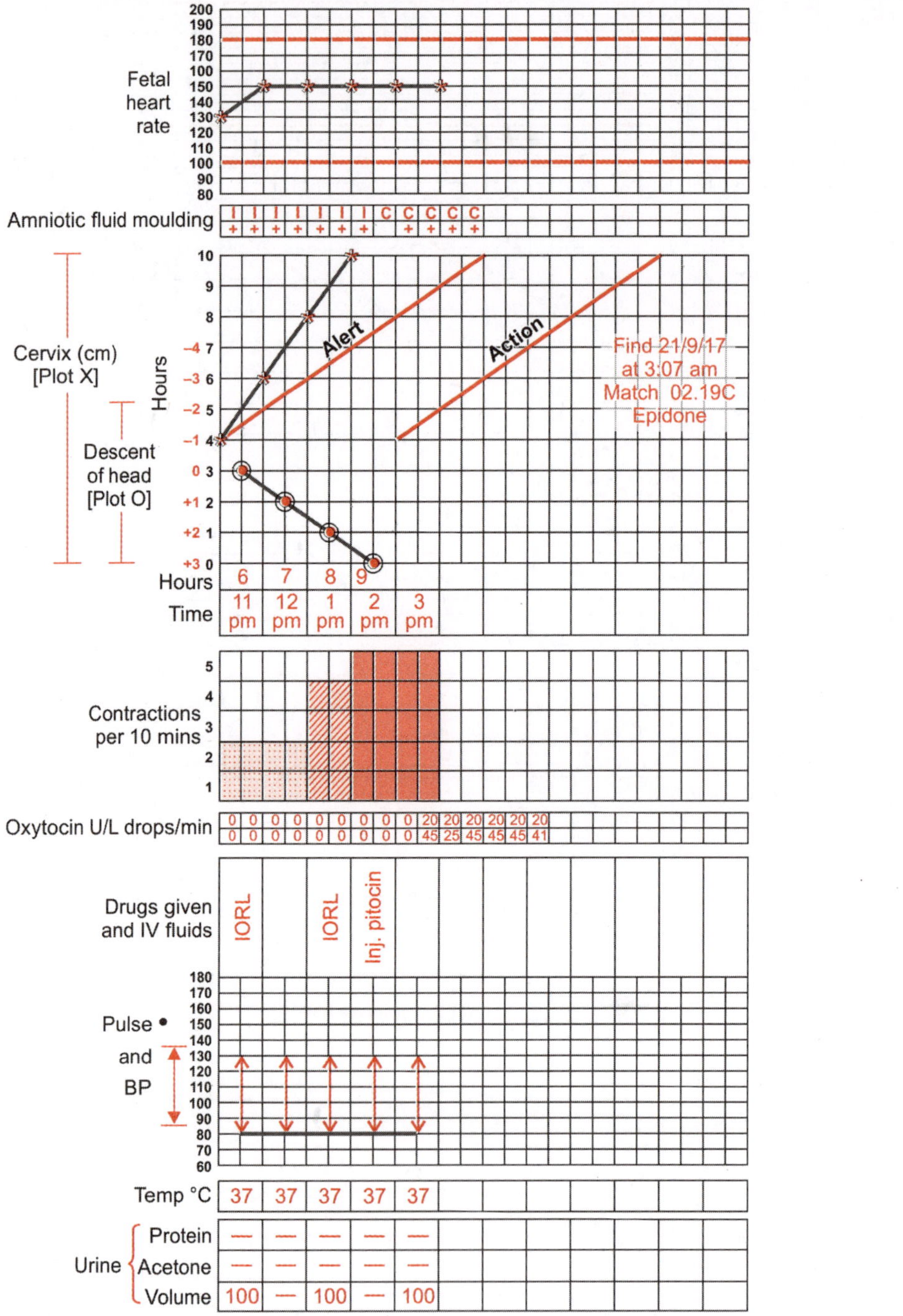
Fetal heart rate
200 190 180 170 100 150 140 130 120 110 100 90 80
Amniotic fluid moulding
I I I I I I I C C C C C
+ + + + + + + + + + +
Cervix (cm) [Plot X]
Hours
Descent of head [Plot O]
10 9 8 -4 7 -3 6 -2 5 -1 4 0 3 +1 2 +2 1 +3 0
Alert
Action
Find 21/9/17 at 3:07 am
Match 02.19C
Epidone
Hours 6 7 8 9
Time 11 pm 12 pm 1 pm 2 pm 3 pm
Contractions per 10 mins
5 4 3 2 1
Oxytocin U/L drops/min
0 0 0 0 0 0 0 0 0 20 20 20 20 20 20
0 0 0 0 0 0 0 0 0 45 25 45 45 45 41
Drugs given and IV fluids
IORL
IORL
Inj. pitocin
Pulse •
and
BP
180 170 160 150 140 130 120 110 100 90 80 70 60
Temp °C 37 37 37 37 37
Urine
Protein — — — — —
Acetone — — — — —
Volume 100 — 100 — 100

CONDUCTING NORMAL DELIVERY

Purposes

- Give comfort, relieve pain, conserve strength, and prevent exhaustion, injury and blood loss
- Maintain cleanliness and asepsis throughout labor
- Carryout careful observation
- Detect deviations from the natural course
- Prevent labor complications
- Recognize complications early and relieve promptly and competently.

Equipments Needed

A sterile tray containing the following articles **(Fig. 7)**:

- Gloves – 2 pairs
- Small bowl containing diluted Savlon
- Small bowl containing normal saline
- Sponge-holding forceps-1
- Gauze pieces
- Draping sheets
- Cotton pads/Sanitary pads-2
- T bandage
- Mopping pads/Sanitary pads 2-3
- Long straight artery forceps-2
- Sterile cotton swabs
- Cord cutting scissors
- Cord clamp
- Mucus sucker
- Blood collection specimen bottles (If required)
- Injection vitamin K
- Kidney tray
- Partograph
- PV examination tray
- Episiotomy and episiotomy suturing tray
- Baby receiving tray with ID band
- Emergency tray containing forceps and vacuum with lubricant

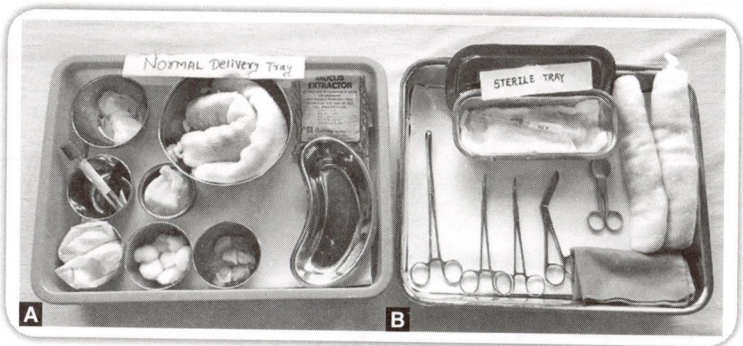

Figs 7A and B: Trays containing articles for normal delivery.
A. Normal delivery tray; B. Sterile tray

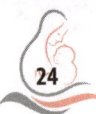

Procedure

Steps of procedure	Rationale
• Receive patient in labor unit once in active phase and maintain partograph timely	• For timely monitoring of patient and notify any deviation from normal
• Provide privacy	• To ensure safe and secure feel for patient
• Perform hand washing before and after each procedure	• To prevent cross infection
• Provide dorsal position with flexed knees to mother once fully dilated	• To enlarge pelvic diameter
• Wear gloves	• To prevent cross infection
• Paint perineum with diluted Savlon and normal saline respectively	• Painting perineum ensures sterility of examination area and prevents ascending infection
• Drape the patient	• To ensures sterility of examination area
• When mother gets contractions, encourage her to hold thighs, take deep breath, close the mouth, hold the breath and bear down or push	• Bearing down at contraction during full cervical dilatation facilitates propulsive and expulsive activities
• When uterine contraction passes off advice mother to open the mouth and take several deep breaths	• Deep breathing during phase of relaxation ensures optimum fetal oxygenation.
• Provide sips of water in between if not contraindicated	• To maintain maternal hydration
• Assistant will support the perineum - paraurethral support by nondominant hand (gauze piece) and rectal support (sanitary pad) by dominant hand	• To prevent perineal injuries
• Give episiotomy at crowning, if required (after anesthetizing by Lignocaine 2%, perineal infiltration)	• To cut short 2nd stage of labor and facilitate safe delivery in case of rigid perineum
• During relaxation apply pressure on the episiotomy	• To minimize bleeding by assuring adequate pressure on active bleeders.
• Deliver head by allowing sinciput to glide slowly over the perineum and allow them to be born till the occiput comes free under the symphysis pubis **(Fig. 8A to F)**	• For smooth and natural delivery

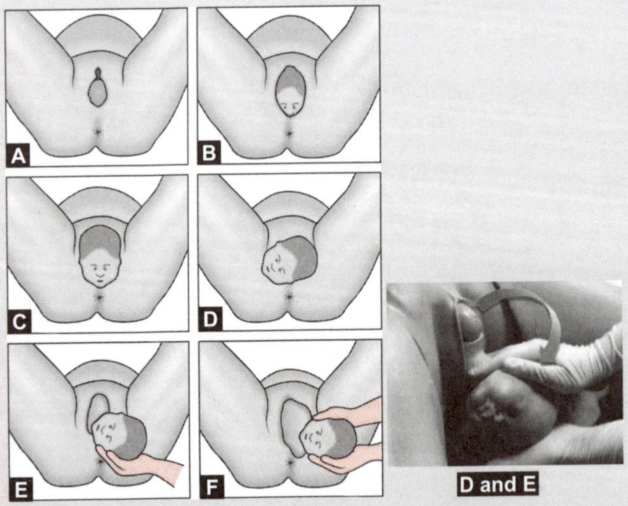

Fig. 8A to F: Delivery of the baby

Contd...

Steps of procedure	Rationale
• Clear eyes with sterile swabs. Suction nose and mouth by mucus sucker	• Eye care to prevent eye infection whereas suctioning to open airway prevent aspiration
• Allow for external rotation of head	• For smooth and natural delivery
• Deliver anterior shoulder then posterior shoulder	• To prevent occlusion of shoulders
• Deliver body by lateral flexion	• For smooth and natural delivery
• Receive baby in baby tray. Clamp the umbilical cord at 5 cm distance from umbilicus and cut the umbilical cord	• For shifting in baby care room
• Dry baby and give tactile stimulation. Monitor APGAR score	• Drying prevents hypothermia whereas tactile stimulation initiates crying reflex in newborn
• Deliver placenta by control cord traction (CCT) after Signs of placental separation like sudden fresh gush of blood, apparent increase in cord length, per abdominally tennis ball like hard uterus, visible fetal part of placenta in introitus	• CCT prevents accidental coed detachment from placenta and uterine prolapsed.
• Deliver placenta in kidney tray and do placental examination	• To ensure complete delivery of placenta and detect placenta-cord anomalies
• Suture episiotomy	• To ensure hemostasis
• Replace all articles	• As per basic principle of good workmanship
• Do recording and reporting	• To ensure SMART documentation

Points to Remember

- • Mother should be comfortable and relax
- • Ensure adequate privacy for mother
- • Have a female attendant compulsory, if delivery is conducted by male candidate
- • Bowel and bladder should be evacuated prior to the procedure
- • Mother should relax and not to contract perineal muscles
- • Give adequate explanation and positive reinforcement during procedure as it is painful.

DELIVERY OF PLACENTA

Purposes

- • To ensure complete delivery of placenta
- • To achieve involution of uterus
- • To reduce chances of retained bits of placenta
- • To achieve hemostasis.

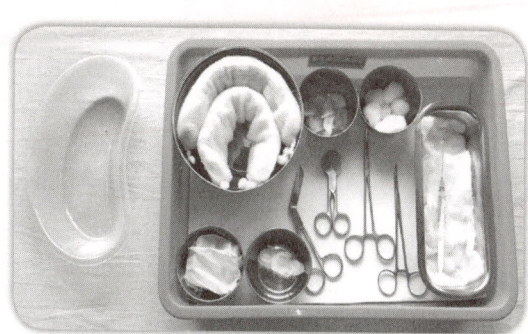

Equipments Needed

A sterile tray containing the following articles **(Fig. 9)**

- • Long artery forceps – 2
- • Umbilical cord cutting scissors – 1
- • Mop

Fig. 9: A tray containing articles for delivery of placenta

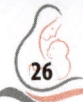

- Kidney tray
- Gloves
- Sponge-holding forceps – 1
- Bowl with Savlon swabs
- Bowl with normal saline swabs
- Sterile pad with T bandage
- Inj Methergine 0.2 mg with 2 mL syringe and Needle 24G, spirit swab (if not contra indicated)

Procedure

Steps of procedure	Rationale
• Placental delivery is done after delivery of baby	• To deliver all product of conception
• Wait for 10–15 minutes after delivery of baby	• To ensure natural separation of placenta
• Wash hands and wear gloves	• To prevent cross infection
• Give dorsal position to patient	• To ensure ease of procedure
• Check the characteristics of uterus	• Contracted and hard uterus indicates placental separation
• Notify signs and symptoms of placental separation ▪ Sudden gush of fresh blood ▪ Apparent lengthening of the cord ▪ Cricket ball like uterus per abdomen ▪ Suprapubic buldge ▪ Feeling placenta per vagina	• Complete delivery of placenta ensures after placental separation
• If these signs and symptoms of placental separation exist hold the cord clamp with right hand and twist round in clockwise direction with gentle traction while give suprapubic pressure with left hand. [(**Control Cord Traction – CCT**) **(Fig. 10A and B)**] **Figs 10A and B:** Guarding the uterus and controlled cord traction	• CCT prevents accidental coed detachment from placenta and uterine prolapse
• When placenta bulges at vagina, hold it with two hands and deliver by rotating it If membranes are threatened to tear they are caught by sponge-holding forceps	• To ensure complete delivery of placenta and prevent retained bits of placenta or membrane
• Give injection Methergine 0.2 mg IM if not contraindicated	• To contract uterus and prevent PPH

Contd...

Steps of procedure	Rationale
• Receive placenta in kidney tray and examine it **(Fig. 11)**	• To detect normal and abnormal placenta/cord.

Fig. 11: Human placenta

Steps of procedure	Rationale
• Remove clots	• To aid in uterine contraction
• Examine perineum for any tear and take corrective actions accordingly	• To detect any tear and take corrective actions accordingly
• Provide perineal care from upward to downward and from inner to outer direction with Savlon and normal saline respectively	• To ensure perineal hygiene and prevent ascending infection
• Tie sanitary pads with T bandage	• For soakage of blood
• Make patient comfortable	• To make patient relax
• Replace all articles	• As per basic principle of good workmanship
• Do recording and reporting	• To ensure SMART documentation

Points to Remember

- Mother should be comfortable and relax
- Ensure adequate privacy for mother
- Only CCT to be followed
- Wait and watch for 10 minutes for signs and symptoms of placental separation
- Avoid fundal pressure, cord pull and unnecessary interventions to deliver placenta
- Examine cord and placenta for any abnormalities
- In case fail to deliver placenta within 30 minutes manual removal of placenta to be done.

EXAMINATION OF PLACENTA

Purposes

- To reduce chances of retained bits of placenta
- To observe placenta and umbilical cord for normal characteristics
- To observe placenta and umbilical cord for abnormal characteristics
- To ensure complete delivery of placenta.

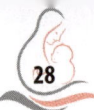
Equipments Needed

A clean tray containing the following articles (**Fig. 12**):

- Mackintosh
- Measuring tape
- Pin (to measure thickness of placenta)
- Cotton tread (to measure diameter of placenta and length of cord)
- Weighing machine
- Gloves
- Kidney tray
- Cotton sab
- Yellow bag

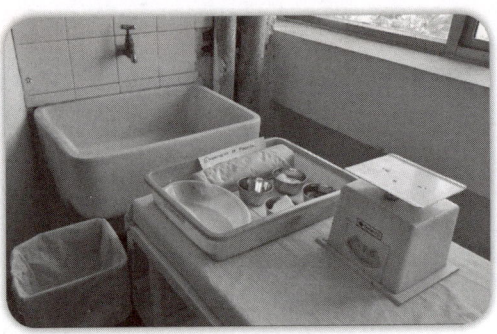

Fig. 12: A tray containing articles for the examination of placenta

Procedure

Steps of procedure	Rationale
• Wash hands and wear gloves	• To prevent cross infection
• Wash placenta under running water	• To remove all clots
• Remove all blood clots	• For better inspection

• **Examination of membranes**
  ▪ Hold the placenta by cord; allow the membranes to hang for easy visualization
  ▪ Insert hand inside through ruptured membranes and visualize membranes
  ▪ Keep placenta on flat surface over mackintosh and examine both surfaces under membranes
  ▪ With cotton swab try to separate amnion from chorion
  ▪ Check for presence of any extra hole in membranes
	• To detect complete/intact delivery of membranes

• **Examination of the placenta**
  ▪ Spread the placenta on palmer aspect of hand or on flat surface for easy visualization (**Fig. 13**)
 	
Fig. 13: Examination of placenta
 	
  ▪ Check the diameter of placenta with thread and measuring tape.
	• To check for normal findings and detect abnormal characteristics

Contd...

Steps of procedure	Rationale
<ul><li>Put pin in the margin and in the center and measure thickness of placenta</li><li>Check fetal surface for the color, appearance, insertion of cord and distribution of the blood vessels (**Fig. 14A**)</li><li>Check maternal surface for number of lobes, color, any calcium deposition or infarcted area (**Fig. 14B**)</li><li>Weigh the placenta</li></ul>	

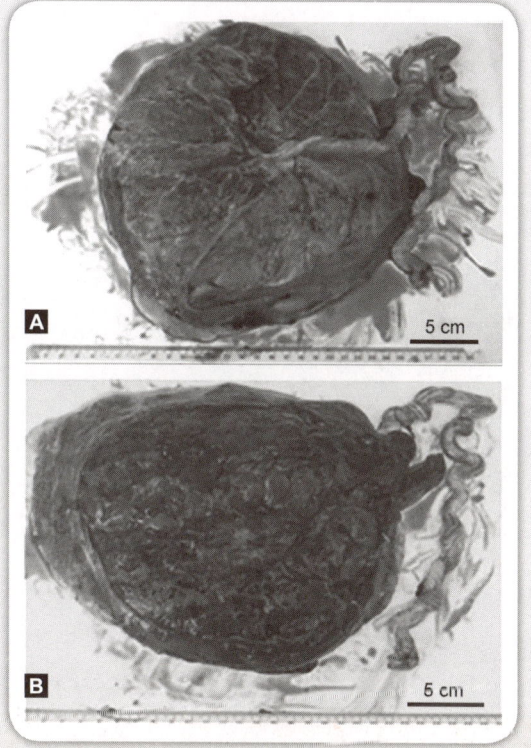

Figs 14A and B: Surfaces of placenta. (A) Fetal side; (B) Maternal side

<ul><li>**Examination of cord**<ul><li>Check for presence of true knots and false knots</li><li>Check the length of umbilical cord</li><li>Check umbilical cord for number of arteries and vein</li></ul></li></ul>	<ul><li>To check for normal findings and detect abnormal characteristics</li></ul>
<ul><li>Replace all articles</li></ul>	<ul><li>As per basic principle of good workmanship</li></ul>
<ul><li>Do recording and reporting</li></ul>	<ul><li>To ensure SMART documentation</li></ul>

Points to Remember

- Do examination after removing all clots
- Examine placenta and cord. Report the findings
- If required label and send it for histopathology

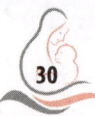

ASSISTING WITH EPISIOTOMY AND SUTURING

Purposes

- To enlarge vaginal introitus
- To reduce second stage of labor
- To minimize overstretching and rupture of perineal muscles
- To facilitate easy and safe delivery
- Delivery of baby in abnormal presentation like breech, face, etc
- As a prerequisite for instrumental delivery (Forceps and vacuum).

Equipments Needed

A sterile tray containing the following articles (**Fig. 15**):

- Gloves
- Bowl with Savlon swabs
- Bowl with normal saline swabs
- Gauge pieces
- Draping sheets
- 10 mL disposable syringe with 21G and 23G needle
- Episiotomy scissors
- Mop
- Needle holder
- Suture material (Chomic Catgut 2-0)
- Toothed thumb forceps
- Sanitary pads with T bandage
- Inj Xylocaine 2%.
- Betadine ointment

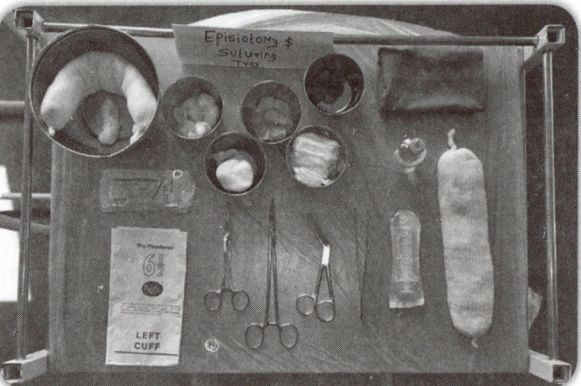

Fig. 15: A tray containing articles for episiotomy and suturing

Procedure

Steps of procedure	Rationale
• Give lithotomy position to patient	• To ease the procedure
• Provide privacy to patient	• To ensure safe and secure feel for patient
• Perform hand washing	• To prevent cross infection
• Wear gloves aseptically	• To prevent cross infection
• Paint perineum from upward to downward and from inner to outer direction with Savlon and normal saline respectively	• As per principle of microbiology clean to unclean. Painting perineum ensures sterility of examination area and prevents ascending infection
• Injection Lignocaine 2% perineal infiltration given in fan fashion	• To ensure adequate anestheting effect
• Place two fingers of left hand (middle and index) in vagina between presenting part and posterior vaginal wall	• To prevent any injury to fetus and for guiding incision
• The incision is made by an episiotomy scissors, blunt blade of which is placed inside, in between the fingers and the posterior vaginal wall and the other on the skin	• To prevent injury to part of presentation

Contd...

Steps of procedure	Rationale
• Incision should be made when Crowning occurs at peak of contraction. Deliberate cut should be made starting from the center of the fourchette extending diagonally either to the right or left (mediolateral episiotomy) (**Fig. 16**)	• To minimize bleeding as crowning thins perineum

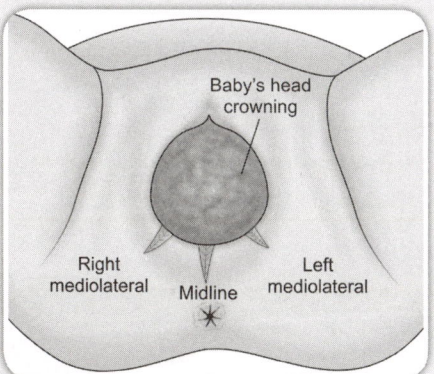

Fig. 16: Types of episiotomy

• It is directed diagonally in a straight line which runs about 2.5 cm away from anus	• Diagonal incision prevents rectal extension
• Deliver baby	• To ensure safe delivery
• Deliver placenta by control cord traction	• To ensure complete delivery of placenta andprevent retained bits of placenta or membrane
• Episiotomy repair is done soon after expulsion of placenta	• To ensure hemostasis and prevent infection
• Mop the perineum and introitus	• To watch for bleeding
• Apex is identified and 1st stitch is taken 0.5–1 cm above the apex (**Fig. 17**)	• To ensure effective hemostasis

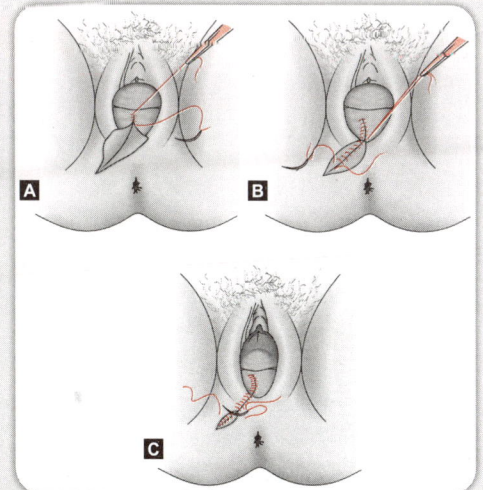

Figs 17A to C: Suturing of Episiotomy episiotomy in three layers. (A) Vaginal mucosa; (B) Muscle layer; (C) Skin

Contd...

Steps of procedure	Rationale
• Apex, vaginal mucosa and submucosal tissues sutured in continuous and interlocking manner	• To ensure adequate hemostasis
• Perineal muscles sutured in intermittent manner	• To ensure adequate hemostasis
• Skin and subcutaneous tissues sutured in mattress and reverse mattress manner	• For better approximation
• Provide episiotomy care and tie sanitary pads with T bandage	• Episiotomy care prevent infection and sanitary pads for blood soakage
• Make patient comfortable	• To relax patient
• Replace all articles	• As per basic principle of good workmanship
• Do recording and reporting	• To ensure SMART documentation

Points to Remember

- Mother should be comfortable and relaxed
- Ensure adequate privacy for mother
- Have a female attendant compulsory, if examined by male candidate
- Mother should relax and not to contract perineal muscles
- Give adequate explanation and positive reinforcement during procedure as it may be painful
- Provide perineal care
- Watch for bleeding

ASSISTING WITH LOWER SEGMENT CESAREAN SECTION

Purposes

- To conduct delivery in case normal vaginal delivery contra indicated.
- To conduct delivery in case of medical, obstetrical complications.
- To conduct delivery when normal or instrumental delivery fails.
- To facilitate easy and safe delivery.

Equipments Needed

A sterile tray containing the following articles (**Fig. 18**):

- Gloves 3–4 pairs
- Bowl with Savlon
- Bowl with normal saline
- Bowl with betadine
- Gauze piece in bundle – 5 bundles
- Sponge holder – 3
- Drapes
- Towel clip
- BP handle No 3 and 4
- Blade no 10 and 20
- Doyen's retractor
- Small retractors – 2
- Toothed forceps – 1

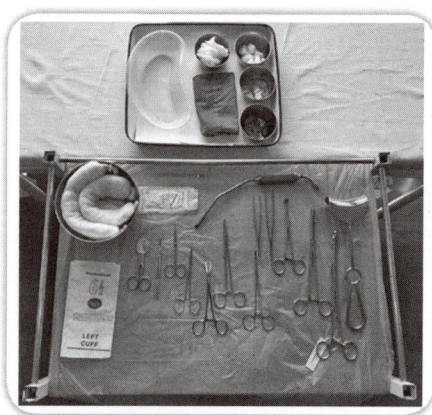

Fig. 18: Tray containing articles for lower segment cesarean section

- Plain forceps – 1
- Tissue cutting scissors – 1
- Mosquito curved artery – 6
- Curved artery forceps – 6
- Green armytage - 6
- Alli's forceps (big + small) – 2 + 4, Total 6
- Babcocks – 2
- Needle holder – 1
- Umbilical cord cutting scissorrs – 1
- Suture cutting scissors – 1
- Suction tube

Procedure

Steps of procedure	Rationale
Pre procedure • Informed consent (surgical, anesthesia, high risk, etc.) • Bowel is emptied with enema at night before or in the morning • Shaving of back, abdomen perineum till mid thigh done • Removal of artificial dentures, earrings, necklace, hair pins, etc • Removal of cosmetics like nail paint, lipstick, etc • Premedication as per prescription • Check for file documentation and all required investigations • Nothing by mouth (NBM) status • Foley's catheterization • Education and counseling of patient and family members about lower segment cesarean section (LSCS) • Confirm operation theater (OT) call • Give sterile cloths with cap to patient and shift to OT	• For legal preparation • To evacuate bowel • To prevent infection • To prevent lost or misplacement of patient belongings. • To detect cyanosis or any other color change at early • To ensure right medication • To ease checking the values/results during procedure • To decrease gastric reflux • To evacuate bladder • For psychological preparation of patient and family • For preventing any delay • To prevent any cross infection

During procedure
• Receive patient in OT
• Assess OT checklist
• Assisting during spinal anesthesia procedure
• Give dorsal position to patient
• Painting of surgical site
 	
• A transverse incision is made about 2 fingers above the symphysis pubis. The anatomical layers incised are (**Figs 19 and 20**):
  ▪ Skin
  ▪ Fat
  ▪ Rectus sheath
  ▪ Muscle (Rectus abdominas)
  ▪ Abdominal/Pelvic peritoneum
  ▪ Uterine muscles.
	• For operative interferences
	• To check for requirements
	• To ensure adequate anesthesia
	• For ease of procedure
	• To ensure sterility of procedure area and prevent ascending infection
	• To ensure adequate incision

Contd...

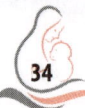
Steps of procedure	Rationale
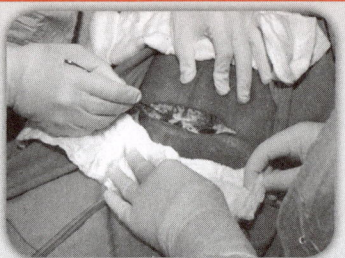**Fig. 19:** Incision to abdominal wall 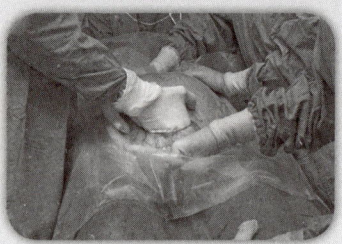**Fig. 20:** Extension of incision • Scrub nurse does mopping in-between and provides required instruments to surgeon. Muscle layer is retracted by small C shape retractors • After incising rectus sheath bladder is retracted by Doyen's retractor • When uterine cavity is opened immediately suctioning done • Once surgeon delivers baby, assisting nurse receives and hand over it to baby nurse (**Figs 21 and 22**) 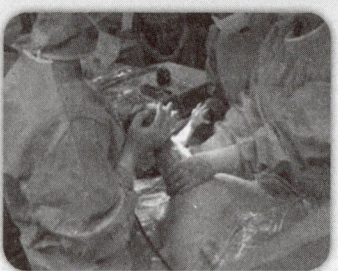**Fig. 21:** Delivery of baby 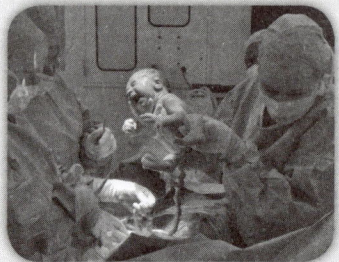**Fig. 22:** Delivery of baby and cord clamping	 • Mopping keeps surgical area clear and free from blood. Retraction required for better visualization • To prevent bladder injury • To clear surgical site and prevent aspiration • To shift baby in baby care room

Contd...

Steps of procedure	Rationale
• Collection of cord blood, if required • After placental delivery examine the placenta • Assist in suturing • Assist in cautery use • Perform count of mop and instruments • Dressing after completion of suturing	• To send for laboratories. • To assess it for normal and abnormal characteristics • To ensure proper closure of incision • To ensure hemostasis • To prevent any lost or misplacement • To maintain sterility of wound
After procedure • Replace all articles • Assess vital signs, AG of patient • Assess for any postsurgical complications • Do recording and reporting	• As per basic principle of good workmanship • To obtain baseline data and see for any deviation. AG to rule out abdominal distension • To see for any deviation and treat accordingly • To ensure SMART documentation

Points to Remember

- Explain procedure to patient and take consent.
- Check for surgical fitness of mother
- Fill OT checklist
- Confirm OT call and shift patient
- Observe patient post procedure to detect any complications early.

ASSISTING WITH FORCEPS/VACUUM DELIVERY

Purposes

- To cut short second stage of labor.
- To fasten delivery in fetal distress.
- To prevent intracranial haemorrhage in case of prematurity (forceps).
- Prolong second stage of labor.

Equipments Needed

A sterile tray containing the following articles (**Fig. 23**):

- Gloves – 2 pairs
- Small bowl containing diluted savlon
- Small bowl containing normal saline
- Sponge-holding forceps – 1
- Gauze pieces
- Draping sheets
- Cotton pads/Sanitary pads – 2
- T bandage
- Mopping pads/Sanitary pads 2–3
- Long straight artery forceps – 2
- Sterile cotton swabs
- Cord cutting scissors
- Cord clamp
- Mucus sucker

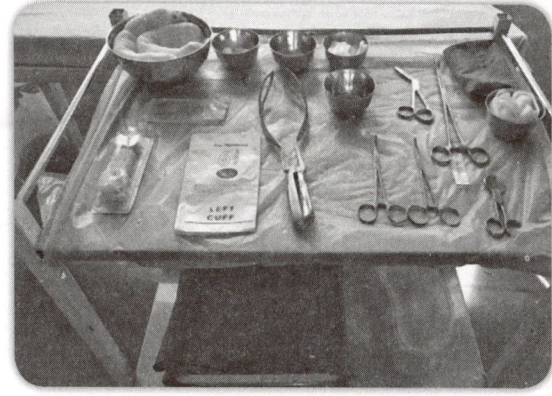

Fig. 23: A tray containing forceps

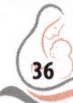
- Blood collection specimen bottles (If required)
- Injection Vit K
- Kidney tray
- Partograph
- PV examination tray

Episiotomy and Episiotomy Suturing Tray

- Tray with forceps/vacuum within different size of cups, lubricant
- Emergency tray containing forceps and vacuum with lubricant **(Fig. 24A and B)**

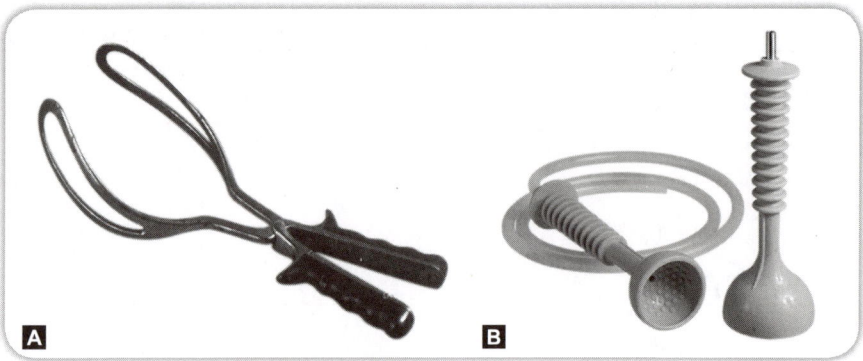

Figs 24A and B: (A) Forceps; (B) Vacuum

Procedure

Steps of procedure	Rationale
• Receive patient in labor unit once in active phase and maintain Partograph timely	• For timely monitoring of patient and notify any deviation from normal
• Provide privacy	• To ensure safe and secure feel for patient
• Perform hand washing before and after each procedure	• To prevent cross infection
• Provide dorsal/lithotomy position to mother once fully dilated	• To enlarge pelvic diameter
• Wear gloves	• To prevent cross infection
• Paint perineum with diluted Savlon and normal saline respectively	• Painting perineum ensures sterility of examination area and prevents ascending infection
• Drape the patient	• To ensures sterility of procedure area
• When mother gets contractions, encourage her to hold thighs, take deep breath, close the mouth, hold the breath and bear down or push	• Bearing down at contraction during full cervical dilatation facilitates propulsive and expulsive activities
• When uterine contraction passes off advice mother to open the mouth and take several deep breaths	• Deep breathing during phase of relaxation ensures optimum fetal oxygenation
• Provide sips of water in between if not contraindicated	• To maintain hydration

Contd...

Steps of procedure	Rationale
• Assistant will support the perineum - paraurethral support by nondominant hand (gauze piece) and perineal support (sanitary pad) by dominant hand	• To prevent perineal injuries
• Give episiotomy	• To enlarge introitus in case of instrumental delivery and to cut short 2nd stage of labor
• During relaxation apply pressure on episiotomy	• To reduce bleeding

• **Application of vacuum (Fig. 25):**
  ▪ Use largest possible cup according to dilatation
  ▪ The cup is introduced after retraction of the perineum with two fingers of the other hand
	• To ensure safe delivery without undue prolongation

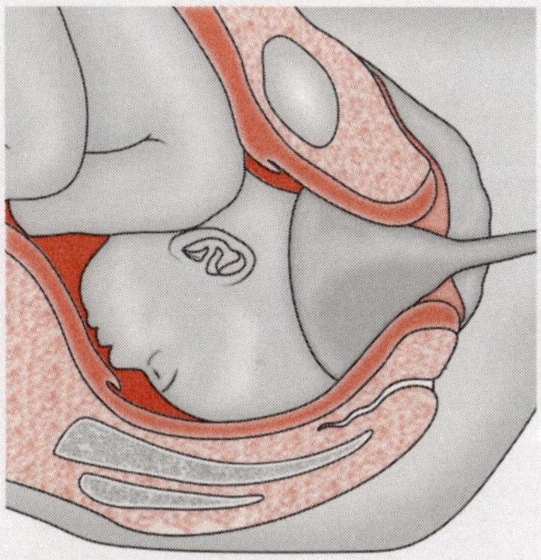

Fig. 25: Application of vacuum cup

- The cap is placed against the fetal head
- Nearer to the occiput with the "knob" pointing toward occiput
- This will facilitate flexion of head and the knob indicates degree of rotation
- A vacuum of 0.2 kg/cm² is introduced by the hand and pumps slowly, taking at least 2 minutes
- Check by using finger rotation around the cup to ensure no cervical or vaginal tissue is trapped inside the cup
- The pressure is gradually raised at the rate of 0.1 kg/cm² per minute until the effective vacuum of 0.8 kg/cm² is achieved in about 3 minutes
- The scalp is sucked into the cup and an artificial caput succedaneum (chignon) is produced
- Traction is provided at right angle to the cup and during uterine contractions in the direction of pelvic axis
- After delivery of head suction machine to be put off the only remove cup
- Deliver shoulder and trunk of baby

Contd...

Steps of procedure	Rationale
• **Application of Forceps (Fig. 26)** 　▪ Prior application, checks blades for correct pair 　▪ Lubricate blades of forceps 　▪ Introduce the left blade of forceps 　▪ Introduce right blade of forceps 　▪ Forceps blades are locked 　▪ Traction is applied with both the hands forward and upward in the direction of pelvic curve 　▪ Provide traction during uterine contractions 　▪ Deliver head, and unlock and remove forceps blades 　▪ Deliver shoulder and trunk of baby	• To ensure safe delivery without undue prolongation

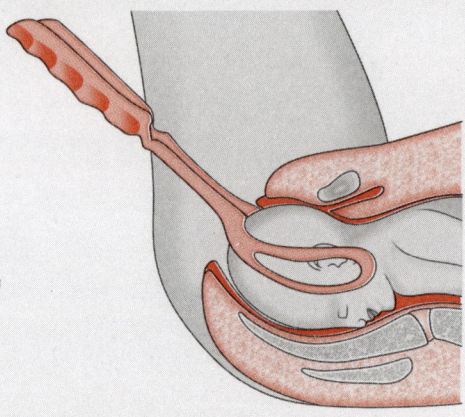

Fig. 26: Application of forceps

Steps of procedure	Rationale
• Clear eyes with sterile swabs. Suction nose and mouth by mucus sucker	• Eye care to prevent eye infection whereas suctioning to open airway preventing the aspiration
• Receive baby in baby tray. Clamp and cut umbilical cord	• For shifting in baby care room
• Dry baby and give tactile stimulation. Monitor **APGAR** score	• Drying prevents hypothermia whereas tactile stimulation initiates crying reflex in newborn
• Deliver placenta by control cord traction (CCT) after signs of placental separation like gush of blood, apparent increase in cord length, per abdominally tennis ball like hard uterus, visible fetal part of placenta in introitus	• CCT prevents uterine prolapse
• Deliver placenta in kidney tray and do placental examination	• To ensure complete delivery of placenta and detect placenta-cord anomalies
• Suture episiotomy	• To ensure hemostasis
• Replace all articles	• As per basic principle of good workmanship
• Do recording and reporting	• To ensure SMART documentation

Points to Remember

- Take second/expert opinion to apply forceps/vacuum
- Explain procedure to patient and take consent
- Mother should be comfortable and relax
- Ensure adequate privacy for mother
- Have a female attendant compulsory, if examined by male candidate
- Mother should relax and not to contract perineal muscles
- Give adequate explanation and positive reinforcement during procedure as it may be painful
- Provide perineal care
- Observe patient postprocedure to detect any complications early.

ASSISTING WITH MEDICAL TERMINATION OF PREGNANCY/ DILATION AND CURETTAGE

Purposes

- To evacuate uterus completely
- To remove all products of conception
- To facilitate involution of uterus
- To send sample for histopathology in recurrent abortion/suspicious products of conception.

Equipments Needed

A sterile tray containing the following articles (**Fig. 27**):

- Gloves 3 – 4 pairs
- Bowl with Savlon
- Bowl with normal saline
- Bowl with betadine
- Gauze piece in bundle – 5 bundles
- Sponge holder – 3
- Drapes
- Towel clip
- Sims speculum
- Vulsellum
- AV retractor
- Dilator set
- Blunt curette
- Ovum forceps
- Suction Cannula set (MVA syringe set) (**Fig. 28**)
- Specimen bottle for histopathology
- Sterile pads with T bandage

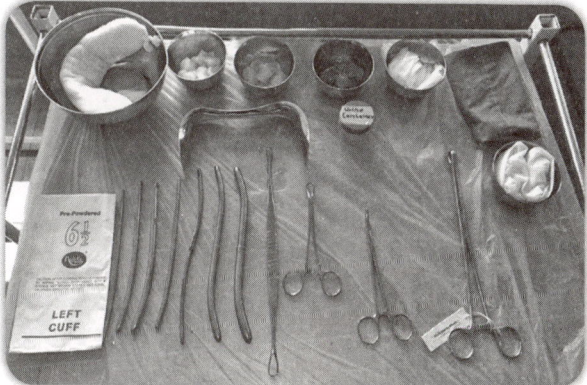

Fig. 27: A tray containing articles for medical termination of pregnancy/dilation and curettage

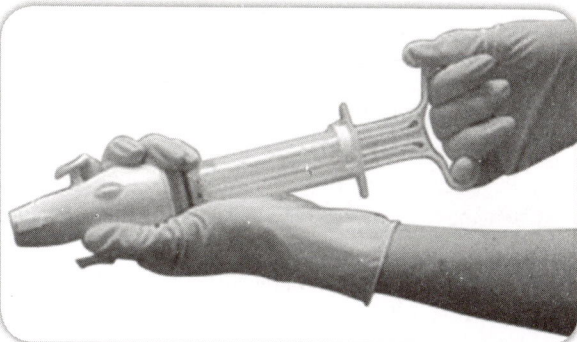

Fig. 28: Vacuum assisted method of D and C

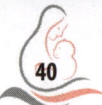
Procedure

Steps of procedure	Rationale
Preprocedure preparation	
• Informed consent. (Surgical, anesthesia, high risk, etc.)	• For legal preparation
• Shaving of abdomen perineum till mid-thigh is done	• To prevent infection
• Removal of artificial dentures, earrings, necklace, hair pins, etc	• To prevent lost or misplacement of patient belongings
• Removal of cosmetics like nail paint, lipstick, etc	• To detect cyanosis or any other color change at early
• Premedication as per prescription	• To ensure right medication
• Check for file documentation and all required investigations	• To ease checking the values/results during procedure.
• Nil by mouth (NBM) status	• To decrease gastric reflux
• Education and counseling, of patient and family members regarding medical termination of pregnancy (MTP)	• For psychological preparation of patient and family
• Confirm OT call	• For preventing any delay
• Give sterile clothes with cap to patient and shift to OT	• To prevent any cross infection
During procedure	
• Receive patient in OT	• For operative interferences
• Assess OT checklist	• To check for requirements
• Assisting during anesthesia	• To ensure adequate anesthesia
• Give lithotomy position to patien	• For ease of procedure
• Perineal painting	• To ensure sterility of procedure area and prevent ascending infection
• Retract posterior vaginal wall with Sims speculum and anterior vaginal wall by AV retractor (**Fig. 29**).	• For clear visualization of cervix

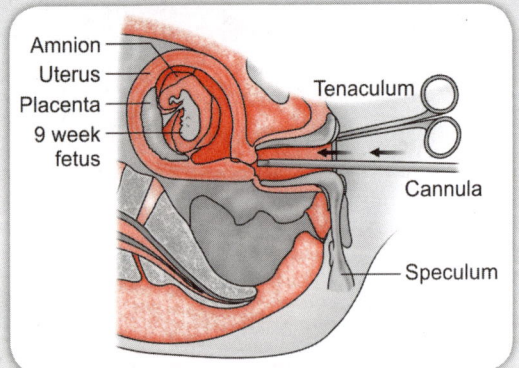

Fig. 29: Cut-away view of mother's pelvis

• Catch and steady cervix with vulsellum/sponge-holding forceps	• To stabilize the cervix
• Start from small number of dilator and increase size gradually	• To dilate cervical of gradually

Contd...

Steps of procedure	Rationale
• Use dilator till number of dilator corresponds to weeks of gestation or weeks of gestation plus 2	• To ensure adequate dilatation
• For dilating pressure/force should be exerted from wrist joint and not from elbow or shoulder	• To prevent any injury
• Dilator has to be held in pen fashion	• To control pressure and avoid excessive force
• Once cervix is adequately dilated use curette for curettage (**Fig. 30**).	• For curretage

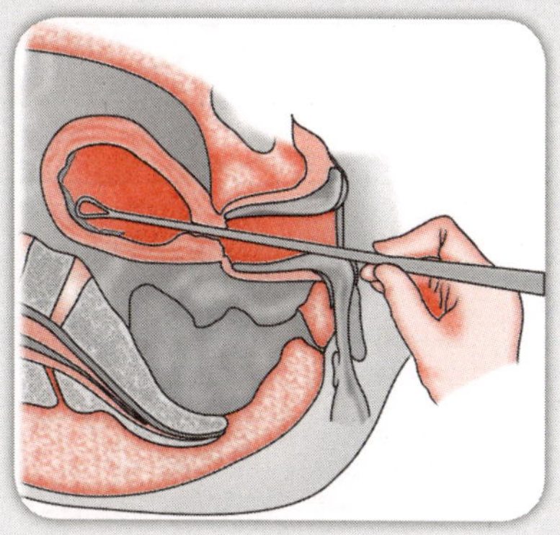

Fig. 30: The uterine cavity is scraped with a curette to determine whether any significant amount of tissue remains.

• Continue curettage till sensation of empty uterus is felt or till bubbling	• To ensure complete evacuation of uterus
• Provide perineal care	• To maintain perineal hygiene
• Make patient comfortable	• To relax patient
After procedure	
• Replace all articles	• As per basic principle of good workmanship
• Assess vital signs of patient	• To obtain baseline data and see for any deviation
• Assess for any postprocedure complications	• To see for any deviation and treat accordingly
• Do recording and reporting	• To ensure SMART documentation

Points to Remember

• Explain procedure to patient and take consent.
• Check for surgical fitness of mother
• Fill OT checklist
• Confirm OT call and shift patient
• Observe patient postprocedure to detect any complications early.

NOTE

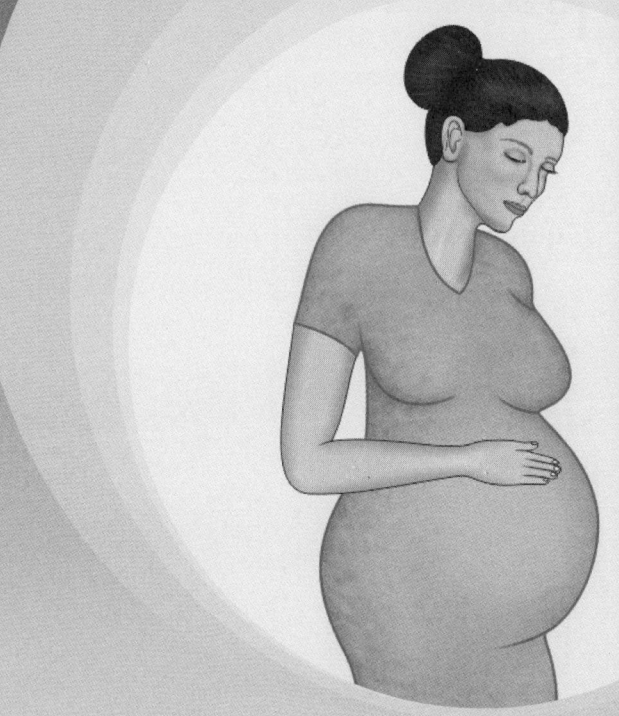

POSTNATAL PROCEDURES

POSTNATAL ASSESSMENT OF THE MOTHER

Purposes

- To assess the health status of the mother
- To detect and treat any complications of mother at the earliest
- To impact family planning guidance.

Equipments Needed

Tray containing the following articles (**Fig. 1**):

- Medium bowl—Warm water to clean the breast
- Small bowl—gauze piece/ cotton swabs
- Measuring tape
- Vital signs tray
- Kidney tray
- Paper bag
- Turkish towel – 1
- Gloves – one pair
- Weighing machine

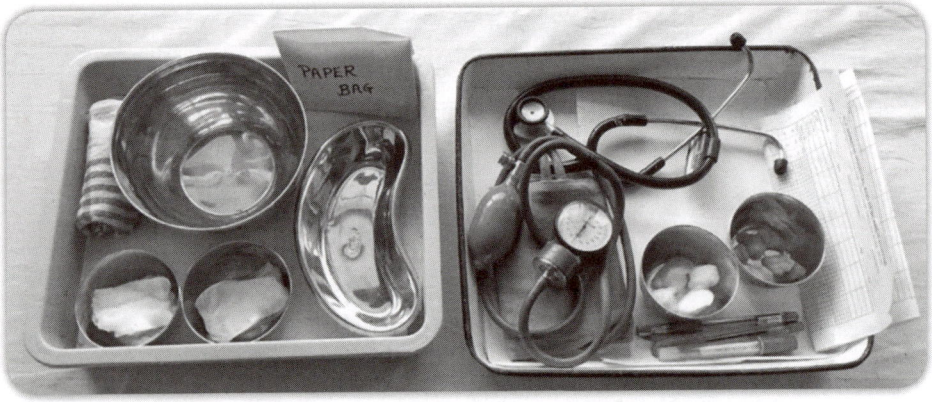

Fig. 1: Tray containing the articles for postnatal assessment

 Mnemonics

POSTPARTUM ASSESSMENT "BUBBLE HE"
B – Breast
U – Uterus
B – Bowel
B – Bladder
L – Lochia
E – Episiotomy
H – Homan's sign
E – Emotional status

Procedure

Steps of procedure	Rationale
• Explain the procedure to the mother	• To get cooperation and avoid anxiety
• Provide privacy with screen	• To ensure safe and secure feel for patient
• Perform hand washing	• To prevent cross infection
• Check the general appearance and vital signs	• To know the base line data
• Perform head-to-toe examination	• To check for any abnormalities
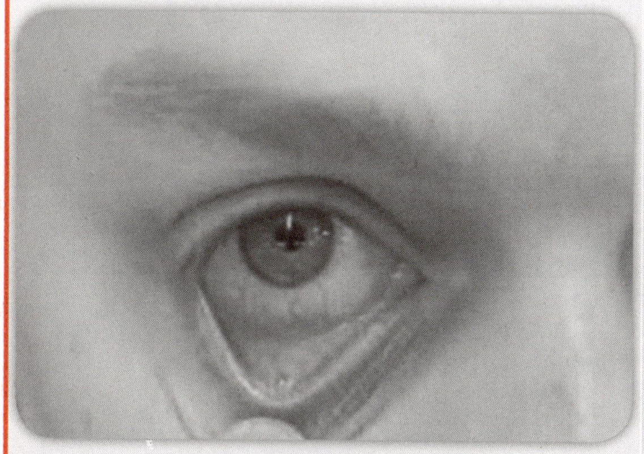 • **Eye:** Pull the conjunctiva downward and observe the lips **(Fig. 2)**	• To look for the pallor and lips for pallor and cracks

Fig. 2: Conjunctival pallor

Steps of procedure	Rationale
• **Breast Examination:** Inspection: expose both the breast	• To look for the symmetry, redness, varicosities and nipples
▪ Observe the nipples for cracked nipples, short nipples, large nipples, inverted and flat nipples	• To maintain hygiene of breast and prevent infection
▪ Clean the breast with warm water and gauze piece in a circular manner and dry it. Repeat to other breast as same manner.	• To identify any tenderness and engorgement
▪ Palpate the breast with any one method (circular, quadrant method, wheel method)	• To easily palpate axilla nodes
▪ Ask the mother to lie on her back with hands under the bed to detect any axillaries nodes	• To avoid unnecessarily exposure and palpate for abnormalities
▪ Cover one breast and palpate the other breast, with finger pads of right hand in a circular motion for any lymph nodes	• To avoid subinvolution
▪ Observe the bladder **and bowel** must be emptied	• Assess for firm/soft/ boggy and contraction
▪ **Abdomen:** Palpate the uterus	▪ To know the process of involution of uterus

Contd...

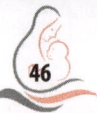

Steps of procedure	Rationale
▪ Assess the involution of the uterus by measuring from the symphysis pubis to fundus of the uterus **(Fig. 3)**	▪ To identify early sign of infection

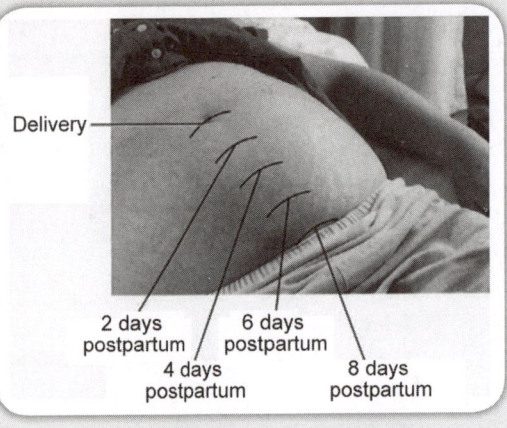

Fig. 3 Assessment of fundal height

▪ Observe the **Lochia** for its types, amount of bleeding and odor and duration **(Fig. 4)**.	▪ To prevent infection

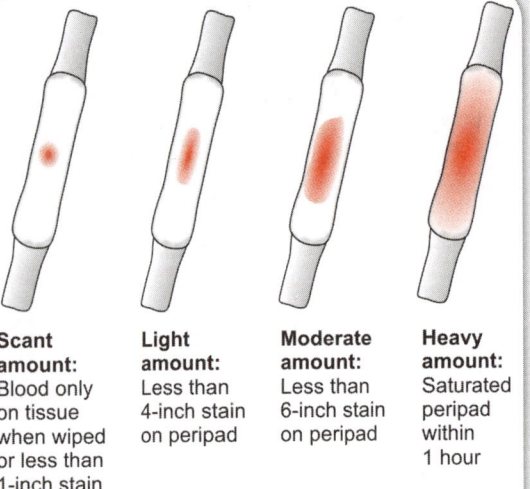

Scant amount: Blood only on tissue when wiped or less than 1-inch stain on peripad

Light amount: Less than 4-inch stain on peripad

Moderate amount: Less than 6-inch stain on peripad

Heavy amount: Saturated peripad within 1 hour

Fig. 4: Assessment of lochia

▪ Observe the **Episiotomy** for **R**edness, **E**dema, **E**cchymosis, **D**ischarge and **A**pproximation **(REEDA)** of the wound	▪ To help in fast healing

Contd...

Steps of procedure	Rationale
▪ Assess the extremities **Homan's sign** deep vein thrombosis (DVT) for varicosities **(Fig. 5)**. Ask the mother to lie on the dorsal recumbent position **Method of Eliciting** Homan's sign, which is characterized by pain in the calf upon dorsiflexion of the foot 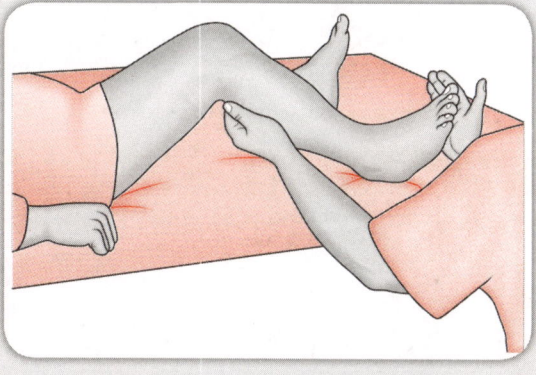 **Fig. 5:** Assessment of Homan's sign	▪ To identify DVT and prevent DVT
▪ Assess the psychological changes of the mother	▪ To ensure mother and baby bonding
▪ Clean and replace the articles	▪ To avoid cross infection
▪ Record and report the abnormal findings (i.e. excessive lochia, foul smelling, subinvolution to the sister/doctor	▪ To notify the physician as soon as possible
▪ Give incidental health education on breast care, breastfeeding and perineal care	▪ To gain knowledge

Points to Remember

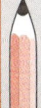

- Mother should be comfortable and relax
- Ensure adequate privacy for mother
- Have a female attendant compulsory, if examined by male candidate
- Bladder should be evacuated prior the procedure
- Notify the doctor for abnormal findings.

BREAST CARE

Purposes

- To clean the breast
- To detect any abnormalities in breast
- To stimulate milk ejection
- To prevent infection
- To prevent breast complications.

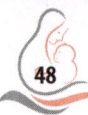

Equipments Needed

- Screen for privacy

A clean tray containing the following articles **(Fig. 6)**:

- Small Turkish towel
- A bowl with 1–2 cotton pads
- A bowl of warm water
- A bowl with cotton swabs to clean the breast
- A bowl with dry gauze pieces to dry the breast
- Kidney tray
- Paper bag

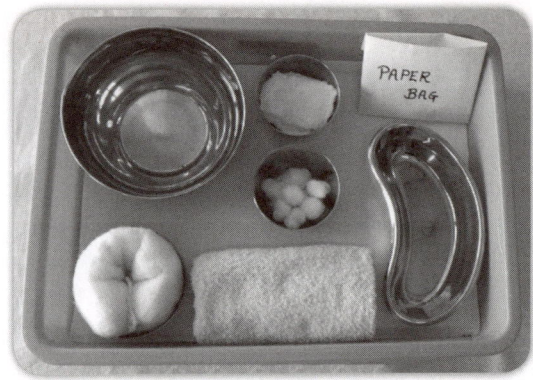

Fig. 6: A tray containing articles for breast care

Procedure

Steps of procedure	Rationale
• Explain the procedure to the mother	• To get cooperation and avoid anxiety
• Provide screen for privacy	• To have a sense of wellbeing
• Provide comfortable position	• To avoid discomfort
• Collect the articles at the bedside	• To avoid interruption between procedure
• Spread the Turkish towel under the patients	• To prevent soiling of linen
• Expose one breast, covering the another breast	• To avoid undue exposure
• **Inspect** the breast	• To see size, symmetry, redness, varicosities and nipples
• Observe the nipples If **cracked nipples**: Wash with clean water and apply emollient **Inverted and flat nipples:** Use the breast pump for expressing breast milk **(Figs 7A to C)**	• To check for cracked nipples, large nipples, inverted nipples and flat nipples

![Types of nipples: A Normal nipple, B Flat nipple, C Inverted nipple]

Figs 7A to C : Types of nipples

• **Short nipples**: Use of pacifier	• To prevent pressure on nipples
• Take the cotton swabs and clean the breast (circular manner) from nipple, primary areola, secondary areola, total breast and lower crease except axilla	• To maintain hygiene and avoid infection

Contd...

Steps of procedure	Rationale
• Take the gauze pieces to dry the breast in the same manner	• To clean the another breast
• Do the same cleaning and drying of another breast in the same manner	• To keep the breast clean and dry
• Palpate the breast with finger pads with any method (Circular, quadrant and wheel method)	• To assess for the tenderness, pain, engorgement and exaggerated lymph nodes
• Squeeze the breast and observe the secretions	• To check for any abnormal secretions
• Clean the secretions with the cotton pads and throw it in the paper bag	• To maintain Hygiene
• Put the baby on breast for feeding	• To enhance proper breastfeeding
• Make the mother and baby comfortable	• To avoid discomfort
• Replace the articles	• To use again
• Record the findings and report for any abnormalities (Tenderness, breast engorgement, mastitis and inverted nipple)	• To notify the physician in early to prevent complications
• Give incidental health education on breastfeeding technique and benefits	• To gain knowledge

Points to Remember

- Mother should be comfortable and relaxed
- Ensure adequate privacy for mother
- Assess the nipple for any deviation from normal and notify to the Physician
- Exclusive breast feeding.

MANUAL EXPRESSION OF BREAST MILK

Purposes

- To express excessive breast milk
- To prevent hardness and engorgement
- To relieve pain
- To enhance proper breastfeeding
- If baby is not able to suck.

Equipment Needed

A clean tray containing the following articles (**Fig. 8**)

- Articles used for breast care (see breast care procedure)
- Small bowl to collect the breast milk

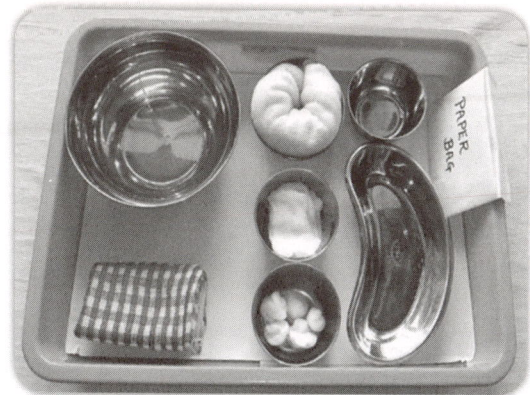

Fig. 8: A tray containing articles for manual expression of breast milk

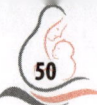

Procedure

Steps of procedure	Rationale
• Explain the procedure to the mother	• To get cooperation from patient
• Provide screen/curtains	• To maintain Privacy of the patient
• Give comfortable position to the mother	• To avoid discomfort
• Perform hand washing	• To prevent cross infection
• Use the **Marmet Technique** Position the thumb (above the nipple) and first two fingers (below the nipple) about 1" to 1–1/2" from the nipple. Be sure the hand forms the letter "C". Avoid cupping of the breast **(Fig. 9A)**.	• To help in proper ejection of breast milk
• Push straight into the chest wall. For large breasts, first lift and then push into the chest wall **(Fig. 9B)**	• To ease ejection of milk from the breast
• Roll thumb and fingers forward at the same time. This rolling motion compresses and empties milk reservoirs without injuring sensitive breast tissue. Note the position of thumb and fingernails during the finish roll as shown in Figure 9C. Repeat rhythmically to completely drain reservoirs. ▪ Position, push, roll….	• To prevent bruising

• **Avoid These Motions**
  ▪ Do not squeeze the breast
  ▪ Sliding hands over the breast may cause painful skin burns
  ▪ Avoid pulling the nipple
	• To prevent tissue damage

• Collect the expressed breast milk in a container **(Fig. 9D)**.	• To preserve or discard the milk
• Repeat the same procedure on the another breast	• To express the breast milk
• Clean and replace the articles	• To maintain cleanliness and later use
• Record the findings and report the abnormality	• Ensure SMART Documentation

Contd...

Steps of procedure	Rationale

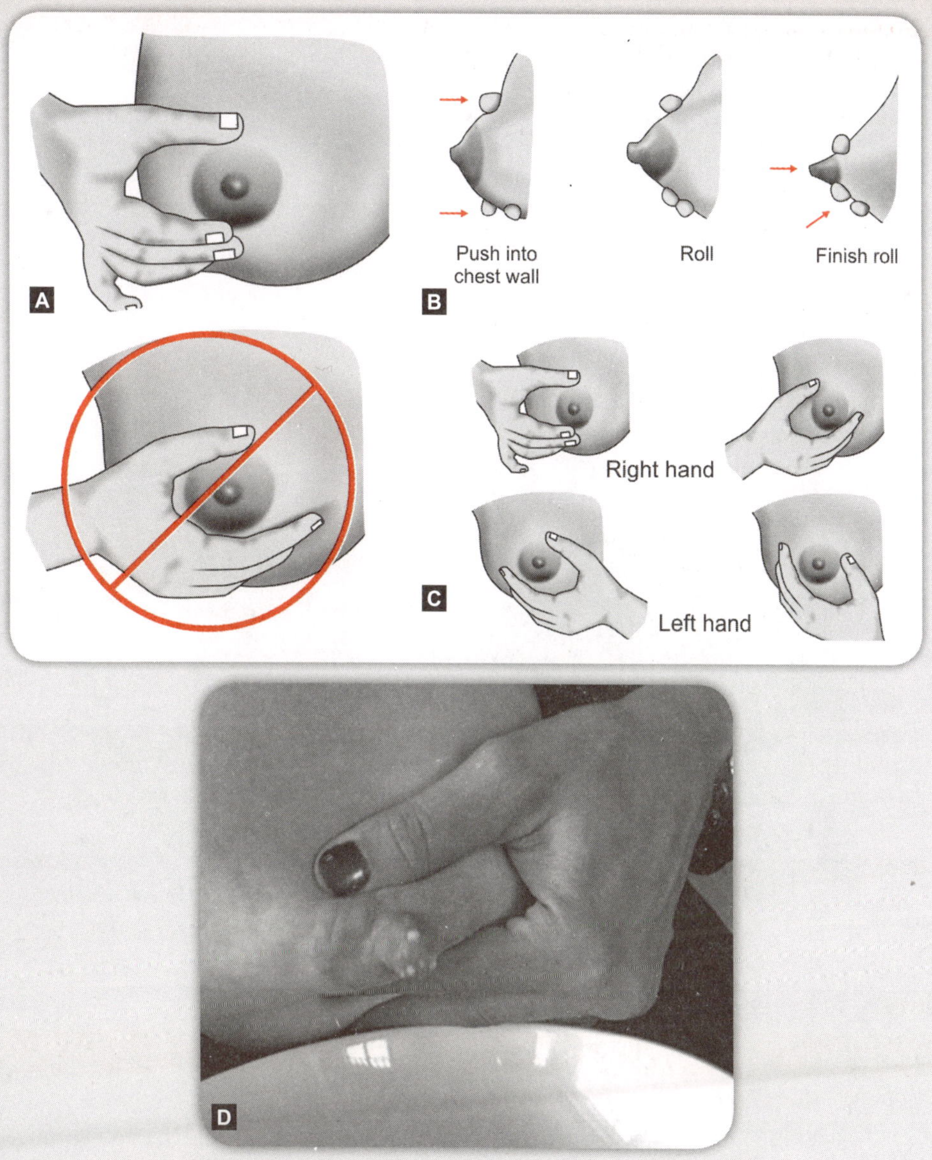

Figs 9A to D: Manual expression of the breast milk Marmet technique

Points to Remember

- Inform the physician for breast tenderness and engorgement
- Inform, if any abnormal findings

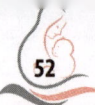
SITZ BATH

Purposes

- It is used to treat hemorrhoids and vaginal fissures
- It promotes healing of episiotomy
- To relieve pain and discomfort
- To reduce swelling and irritation
- To increase circulation
- To promote relaxation.

Equipments Needed

A clean tray containing the following articles (**Fig. 10**):

- Bath tub and shallow bucket
- Potassium permanganate salts (if ordered)
- Warm water ($105°F–110°F$)
- Towel (Gloves, if required)

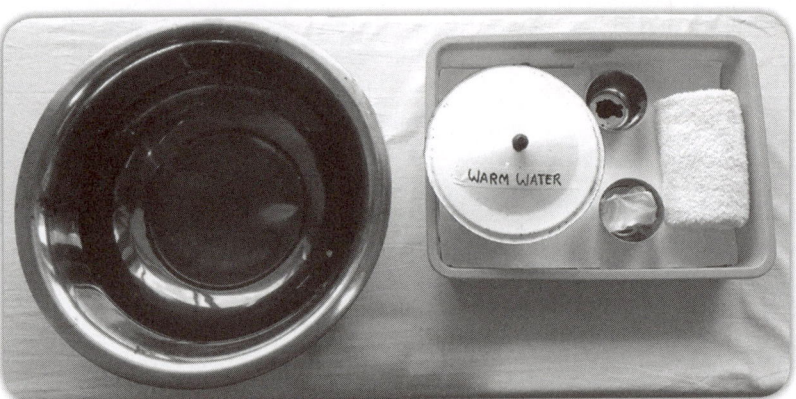

Fig. 10: A tray containing articles for sitz bath

Procedure

Steps of procedure	Rationale
• Provide privacy	• To avoid anxiety
• Fill 3/4th of the tub with warm water	• To Avoid chillness and feel warm
• Can add a pinch $KMNO_4$ salts (till it becomes light pink) if recommended by the physician	• To help in fast healing
• Keep the basin on a low stool	• To drain the extra water
• Place towel on the patients thigh and cover it	• To avoid exposure
• Instruct the patient to contract and relax anal sphincter	• To loosen the perineal muscles

Contd...

Steps of procedure	Rationale
• Encourage the patient to sit in the water for about 20–30 minutes **(Fig. 11)**	• To relieve from pain and reduce swelling

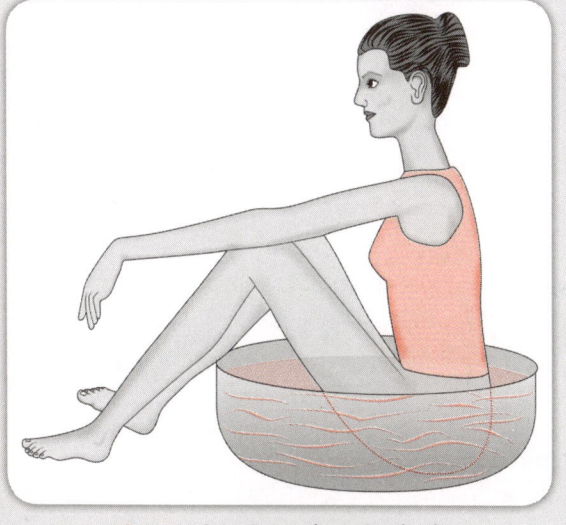

Fig. 11: A patient taking Sitz bath

Steps of procedure	Rationale
• Dry the perineum and apply dressing or peripad	• To avoid microorganisms growth
• Clean and replace the articles	• To avoid cross infection and use for next time
• Recording and reporting	• For SMART documentation

Points to Remember

- Notify the physician for redness, discharge and swelling in perineum
- To assess for any hemorrhoids and fissures.

PERINEAL CARE/EPISIOTOMY CARE

Purposes

- To clean the perineum
- To relieve inflammation
- To relieve pain and stimulate circulation
- To encourage the healing process
- To prevent spread of infection and bacterial growth
- To apply medication over episiotomy wound
- To promote a sense of wellbeing and comfort.

Equipments Needed

- Screen or curtains for privacy

A clean tray containing the following articles (**Fig. 12A**):

- A bowl with warm water
- Betadine ointment or cream
- Sterile sanitary pad – 2 or T binder
- Mackintosh with towel
- Clean gloves- one pair
- Kidney tray
- Paper bag
- Bedpan

A sterile tray containing contacting the following articles (**Fig. 12B**)

- A small bowl with sterile 9–12 cotton swabs soaked in Savlon solution of 1:20 ratio
- A small bowl sterile 9–12 cotton swabs soaked in with normal saline
- A small bowl with sterile 9–12 cotton swabs soaked in a Betadine solution (if required)
- Long artery forceps /sponge-holding forceps– 1
- Dissecting forceps –1
- Bowl with sterile gauze pieces 9–12 to dry the perineum
- Sterile gloves one pair

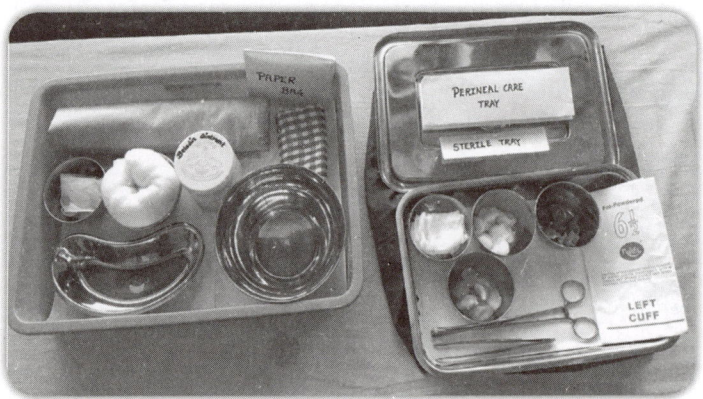

Figs 12A and B: Tray containing articles for perineal care.
A. Clean tray; B. Sterile tray

Procedure

Steps of procedure	Rationale
• Explain the procedure to the mother	• To get cooperation
• Provide privacy by screens	• To maintain privacy
• Make the patient comfortable	• To avoid discomfort
• Collect all the articles	• To save time and energy
• Perform hand washing	• To prevent cross infection

Contd...

Steps of procedure	Rationale
• Give dorsal position, remove the soiled sanitary pad and spread the mackintosh	• For easy cleaning and exposure of perineal area
• Expose the perineum, put the bed pan under and pour the warm water over the perineum	• To clean the soiled area
• Wash hands properly and wear gloves	• To prevent infection
• Clean the stitches of episiotomy first with Savlon give one stroke with sterile forceps and keep it dry	• To remove excessive blood
• Clean the pubic area with Savlon, normal saline and dry with gauze piece with single stroke manner	• To remove excess blood
• Clean the perineum using Savlon cotton swabs with forceps or with gloved hand from above downward in the following order in a **single stroke manner**	• To prevent Infection
• Clean vulva, i.e. (i) Urethra toward anus, (ii) Labia minora– farthest side first then nearest side, (iii) Labia majora inner side – same manner and (iv) Labia majora outer side – same manner (**single stroke manner)**	• Wash from clean to unclean area
• Clean the episiotomy wound in one stroke and squeeze and rotate from up downward	• To check for any discharges and prevent infection
• Clean the episiotomy wound in one stroke and squeeze and rotate from up downward for any discharges	• To clean the excess savlon solution
• Clean the anus thoroughly in a circular motion	• To remove dirts/ blood clots
• Clean the perineum using normal saline cotton swabs in the same manner	• To remove excessive Savlon solution and maintain hygiene
• **If required, use betadine cotton swabs in a same manner**	• If infected (According to hospital protocol)
• Dry the perineum with gauze pieces.	• Drying helps in preventing microorganism growth
• Apply betadine ointment or cream over the episiotomy wound and cover with dry gauze piece	• Helps in fast healing and relieve of pain and swelling
• Apply sanitary pads or T binder and panty	• To prevent soiling
• Remove gloves and replace the articles and make the patient comfortable	• To avoid cross infection and feel sense of wellbeing
• Recording and reporting (REEDA)	• To notify the physician for early signs of complications
• Give incidental health education on perineal care	• To gain knowledge and proper care

Points to Remember

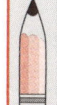

- Check for REEDA Score
- Apply Betadine cream on episiotomy
- Proper hygiene should be maintained.
- If pain, excessive bleeding, wound gaping or purulent excessive discharges, notify the physician

NOTE

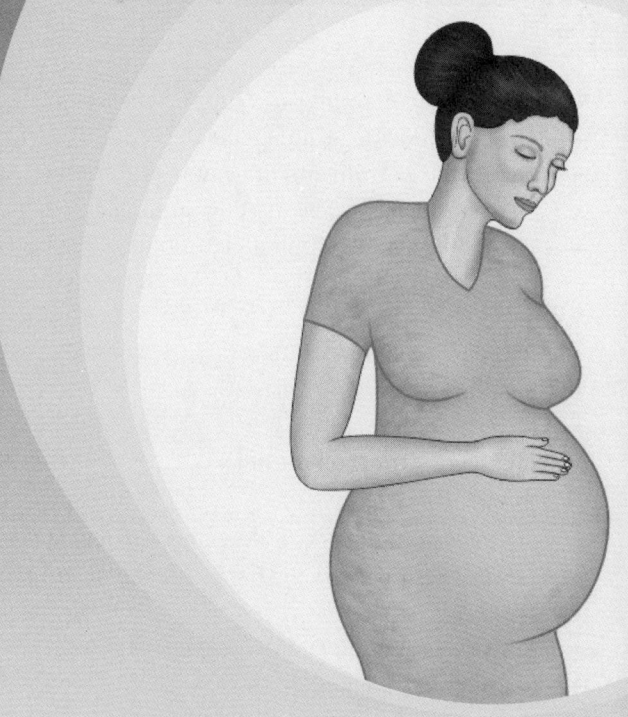

NEONATAL PROCEDURES

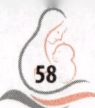

IMMEDIATE NEWBORN CARE

Purposes

- To establish, maintain and support respiration
- To clear air passage and facilitate breathing
- To provide warmth and prevent hypothermia
- To ensure safety, prevent injury and infection
- To identify actual or potential problems that may require immediate attention.

Equipments Needed

- Radiant warmer
- Suction apparatus
- Oxygen apparatus
- Emergency tray consist of (laryngoscope with blade, neonatal mask, Ambu bag and emergency drugs)

A clean tray containing the following articles **(Fig. 1)**

- Dry linen (one to dry the baby and one to wrap the baby)–2
- Head cover–1
- Mucus extractor or suction catheter–1
- Sterile gauze piece–2
- Umbilical cord scissors–1
- Identification tag–1
- Cord clamps–1
- Sterile spirit cotton balls–4
- Baby cloth

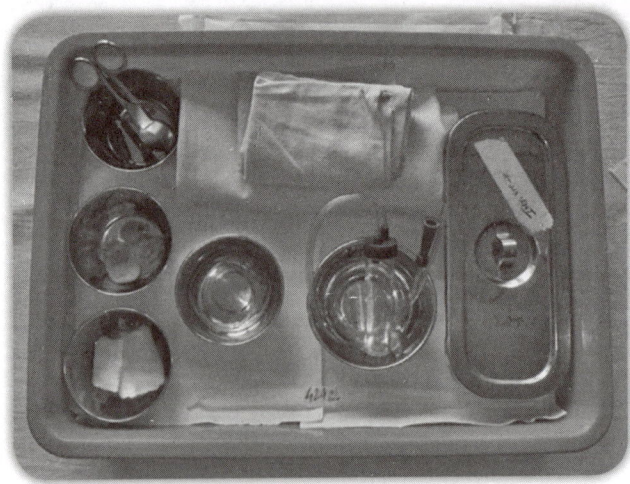

Fig. 1: A tray containing articles for immediate newborn care

Procedure

Steps of procedure	Rationale
• Perform hand washing and wear gloves	• To perform asepsis
• Receive the baby in tray covered with sterile linen with head slightly downward	• To remove excess secretions
• Suction the secretions from mouth and nose by mucus extractor or bulb syringe (suction mouth first, then, the nose (**Fig. 2**).	• To prevent aspiration

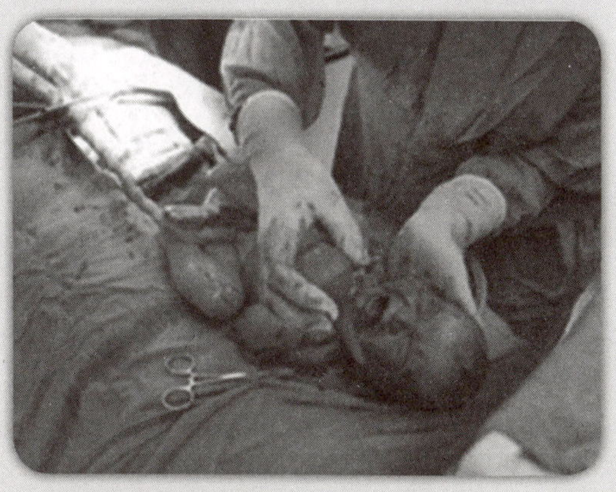

Fig. 2: Section of secretion from mouth by bulb syringe

• Gently wipe the baby eyes with sterile cotton balls and remove the wet linen	• To clean the eyes
• Place the baby in dry linen	• To prevent hypothermia
• Check **APGAR** score at the end of 1 minute, 5 minutes and 10 minutes (**Fig. 3**)	• To know the general condition of baby

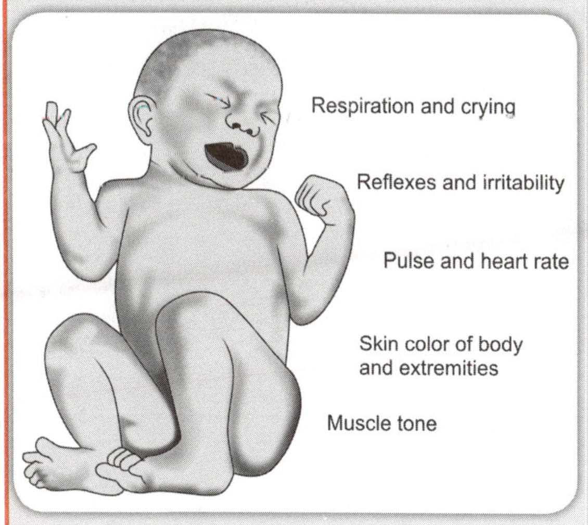

Respiration and crying

Reflexes and irritability

Pulse and heart rate

Skin color of body and extremities

Muscle tone

Fig. 3: Apgar score to measure the physical condition of new born infant

Contd...

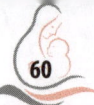
Steps of procedure	Rationale
• Clean the baby	
• Clamp and ligate the cord. Apply cord clamp **(Fig. 4)**	• To prevent bleeding

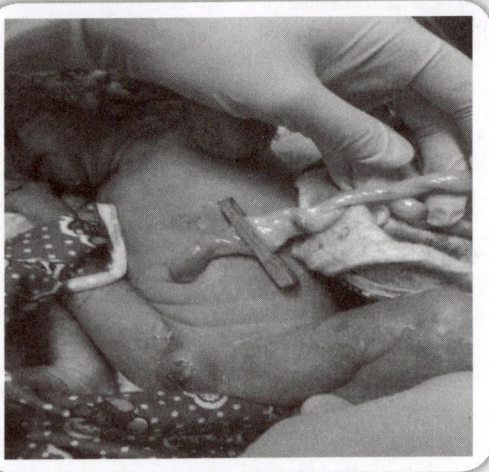

Fig. 4: Cord clamp applied in the cord

• Confirm the gender of the baby to the mother	• To avoid misconceptions of sex of baby
• Weigh the baby **(Fig. 5)**	• To know the birth weight

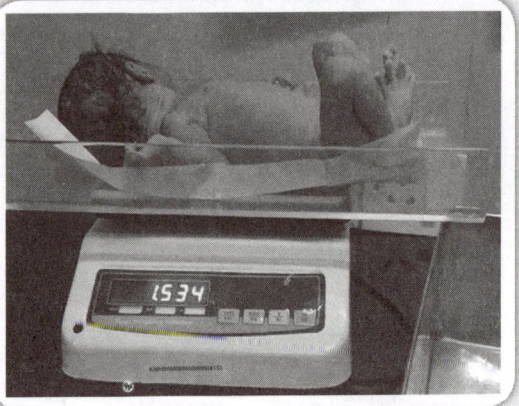

Fig. 5: Weighing the infant

• Tie the identification tag (according to hospital protocol)	• To avoid misplacing of babies
• Observe for any abnormality of the baby	• For early detection
• Take a foot print or photograph with one parent	• For identification of the baby

Contd...

Steps of procedure	Rationale
• Keep the baby under radiant warmer and give injection of vitamin K, 1 mg intramuscular. (**Fig. 6**)	• To prevent hypothermia

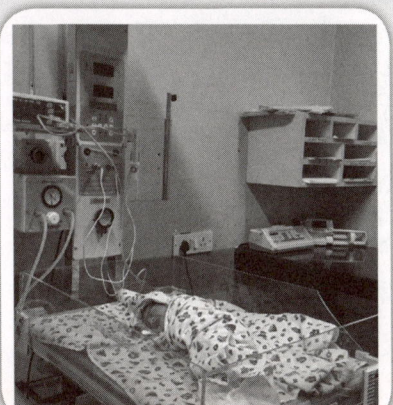

Fig. 6: Baby under radiant warner

Put the head cap and dress.

• Check apgar score	• To assess the general condition
• Recording and reporting	• To ensure smart documentation

Points to Remember

- If Apgar score is below 7 or there are any congenital abnormalities, inform the sister in-charge or physician
- Perform quick check of any abnormalities
- Injection vitamin K should be administered only in recommended dose
- Keep the baby under radiant warmer

NEWBORN ASSESSMENT

Purposes
- To detect any abnormality
- To assess the baby's thermal regulation

Equipments Needed
A tray containing the following articles (**Fig. 7**):
- Cotton swabs to clean the baby
- Torch
- Measuring tape
- Paper and pen to write
- Eye care and cord care tray

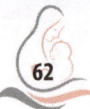
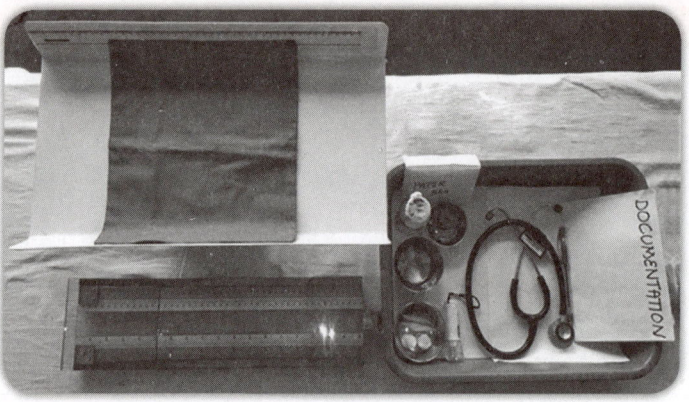

Fig. 7: A tray containing the articles for newborn assessment

Procedure

Steps of procedure	Rationale
• Explain the procedure to the mother	• To get cooperation
• Keep the tray nearby the patient	• To save time and energy
• Switch off the fan	• To avoid hypothermia
• Assess the vital signs—temperature, heart rate, respiration and blood pressure	• To know the general condition
• Assess the anthropometric measurements [weight, length, head circumference, chest circumference **(Fig. 8)**]	• To assess any abnormalities

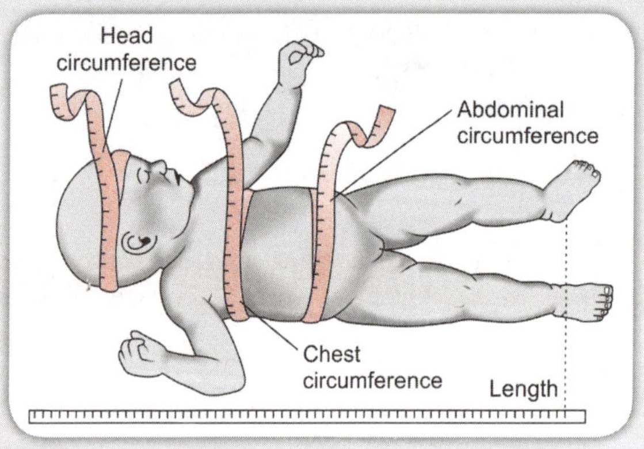

Head circumference

Abdominal circumference

Chest circumference   Length

Fig. 8: Assessment of head circumference, chest circumference, abdominal circumference and length

• Assess the skin for appearance for vernix caseosa, milia, erthyema toxicum, Mongolian spots	• To check for normal physiological changes
• Assess the head for fontanels, caput succedaneum, cephal hematoma **(Fig. 9)**	• To rule out any problem like ophthalmia neonatorum or infection

Contd...

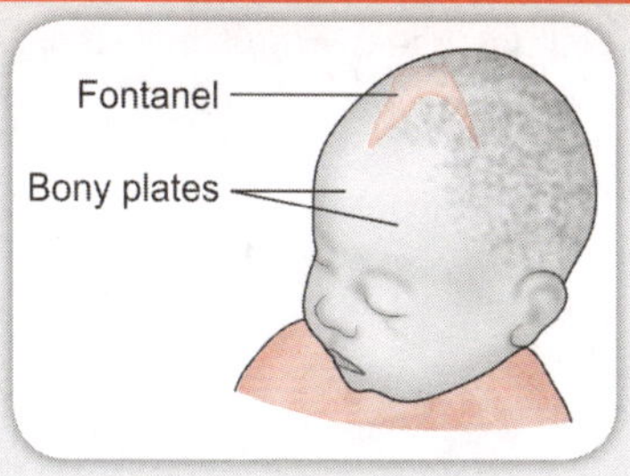

Steps of procedure	Rationale

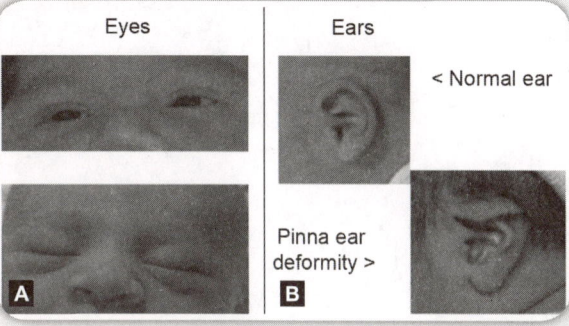

Fig. 9: Physical examinations of head and neck in newborn.

- Assess the face: (a) Observe the **eyes** for symmetry, sclera and symmetry of movement, conjunctiva and iris **(Fig. 10A)**
  - Observe the **ears** for position (drawing an imaginary horizontal line from the inner canthus of the eyes perpendicular to the vertical axis of the head) **(Fig. 10B)**

| | • To check for any Down's syndrome baby |

Figs 10A and B: Physical examination A. Eyes; B. Ears

- Observe for **hearing**: Alertness and stops movement in the presence of conversation or noise
- Observe the **nose** for symmetrical, patent and deviation
- Observe the **mouth**

| | • To check the hearing capacity

• For patency or any nasal deviation

• To rule out for cleft lip and cleft palate, deciduous teeth, oral thrush |

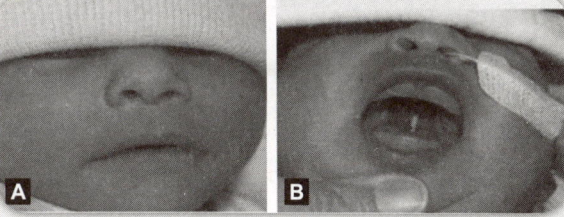

Fig. 11A and B: Physical examination A. Nose; B. Mouth

- Observe the **chin**
- Assess the **chest**
- Assess the **abdomen**

| | • To rule out for open at equal angles bilaterally
• For shape, symmetry, nipple discharge
• For softness |

Contd...

Steps of procedure	Rationale
• Assess the **umbilicus (Figs 12A and B)**	• For redness, infection and dryness of cord

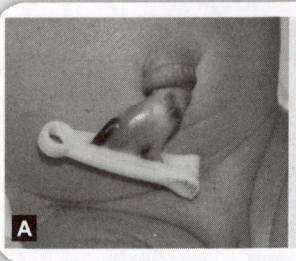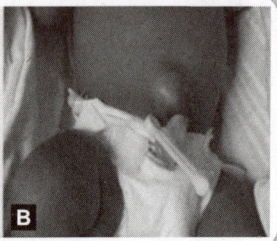

Fig. 12A and B: Physical examination of the umbilicus. A. Normal; B. Umbilical hernia

• Assess the **genitalia and anus (Figs 13A to F)**
  ▪ Female in term baby for labia majora, covers the labia minora (in preterm baby for clitoris is prominent) vaginal opening patent and discharge.
  ▪ Male for the gland is completely covered by foreskin at birth. Penis length, testes for descended, scrotum is highly pigmented
  ▪ Anus and rectum
	• To rule out any abnormalities
	
	• For patency, imperforated anus

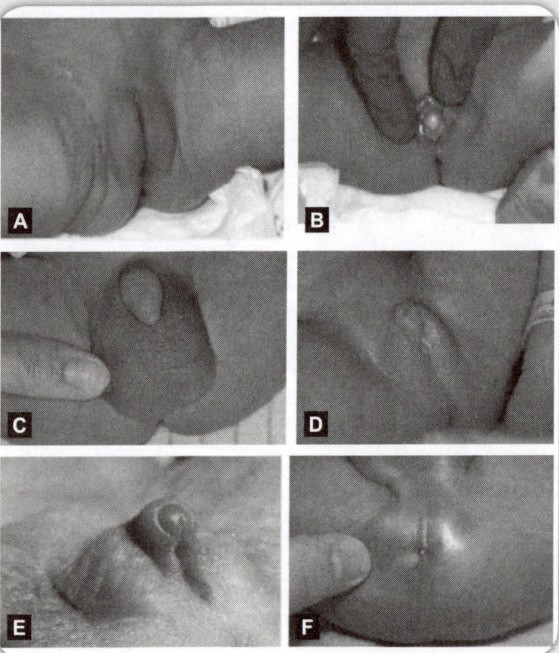

Fig. 13A to F: Physical examination of genitalia in newborn baby. A. Normal female genitalia; B. Abnormal female genitalia; C, D Male genitalia for any abnormality; E. Ambiguous genitalia; F. Closed rectum

Contd...

Steps of procedure	Rationale
• Assess the **musculoskeletal system.**	• For spine for normal curvature, posture, spina bifida and meningomyelocele
• Assess the **central nervous system** for reflexes.	• To rule out any abnormal reflexes
• Recording and reporting the abnormal findings.	• To notify the doctor early signs and symptoms

Points to Remember

- • Maintain thermoregulation
- • Handle the baby gently
- • Do not over stimulate the baby.

EYE CARE

Purposes

- To clean the secretion
- To protect from infection

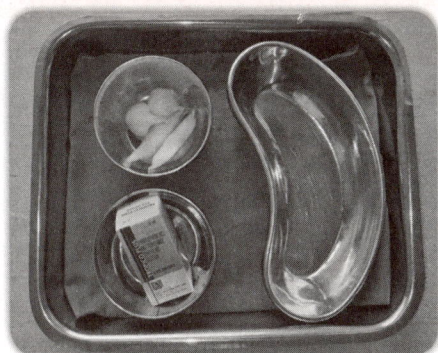

Equipments Needed

A sterile tray contains the following articles **(Fig. 14)**

- Cotton swabs soaked with warm sterile water
- Kidney tray
- Eye drops or ointment, if required

Procedure

Fig. 14: A trey containing articles for eye card

Steps of procedure	Rationale
• Wash the hands properly	• Maintain aseptic measures
• Take a soaked sterile swab and squeeze the excess water	• To avoid spilling
• Clean from medial to lateral side or inner canthus to outer canthus one stroke	• Less contaminated to more contaminated areas to avoid infections
• Repeat the other eye in same manner	
• Apply eye drops or ointment if prescribed (from inner canthus to outer canthus) if infected, apply drops/ointment in the clean eye first and then in the affected eye) **(Fig. 15)**	• To prevent infection

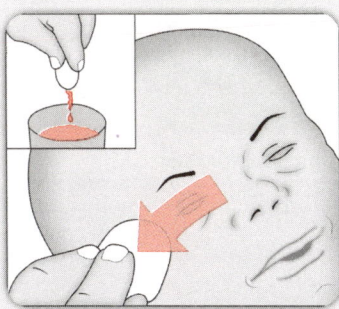

Fig. 15: Performing care of the eye of a newborn

Contd...

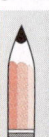

Steps of procedure	Rationale
• Do not apply anything else (e.g. kajal) in the eyes	• To prevent eye infection
• Clean and replace the articles	• To avoid cross infection
• Recording and reporting (any signs of infection)	• To detect abnormalities early

Points to Remember

- Avoid spreading of cross infection
- Clean form inner canthus to outer canthus
- Powdered gloves are not allowed during the procedure.

UMBILICAL CORD CARE

Purposes

- Keeping the umbilical cord stump clean and dry is important. This helps to prevent infection and irritation
- It may also help the stump to fall off and the navel heals quickly
- In general, one can keep the stump clean by leaving it alone.

Equipments Needed

Clean tray containing the following articles **(Fig. 16)**
- Gauze piece/cotton
- Spirit/betadine/normal saline as per hospital protocol
- Kidney tray

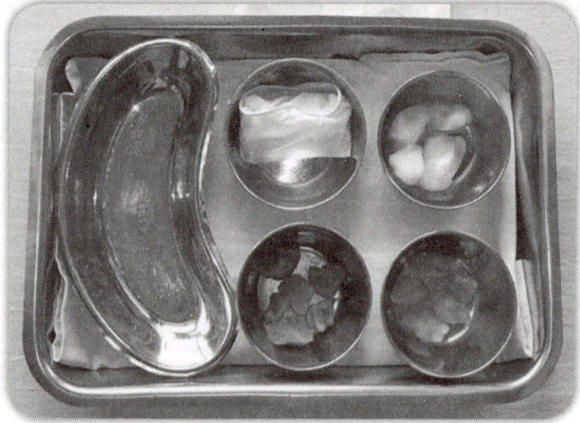

Fig. 16: A tray containing articles for umbilical cord care

Procedure

Steps of procedure	Rationale
• Wash the handle properly	• To prevent infection
• Observe the umbilical cord	• Assess for sign of drying for any redness, discharge, (dirty or sticky)
• Get a gauze piece soaked with any one of the solutions	• To clean the cord
• Clean the skin surrounding area of the umbilical cord 1st stroke outer to inner, 2nd stroke to umbilical stump in a circular manner and 3rd stroke above the clamp (Fig. 17) 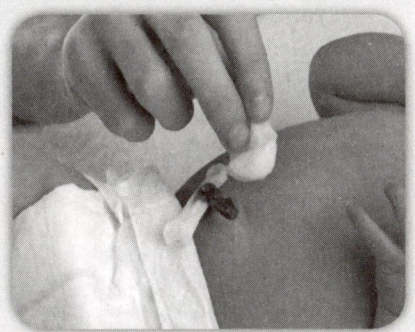 **Fig. 17:** Cleaning the skin surrounding area of the umbilical cord	
• Repeat with Betadine as same manner	• To prevent infection
• Dry the stump by holding a clean cloth or dry gauze around it	• Moisture leads to growth of microorganisms
• To clean the umbilical cord stump once each day until it falls off	• For fast drying
• Exposing the stump to air helps it to dry out and fall off	• Helps in fast drying
• Recording and reporting (any sign of infection, i.e. redness, oozing, etc.)	• To detect early complications
• Replace the articles	

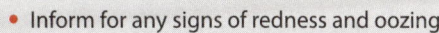

Points to Remember

• Inform for any signs of redness and oozing
• Do not apply any ointment
• Do not put tight clothing or diaper on cord (Fig. 18).

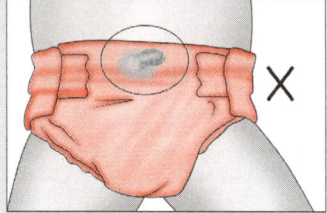
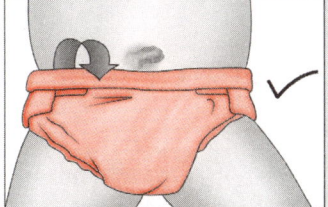

Fig. 18: Correct-method of putting cloth diaper

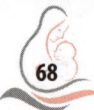
MOUTH CARE

Purposes

- To keep the mouth of the baby clean
- To prevent oral thrush or any infection

Equipments Needed

A clean tray containing the following articles (**Fig. 19**):
- Piece of gauze and cotton or cloth
- Glass of drinking water

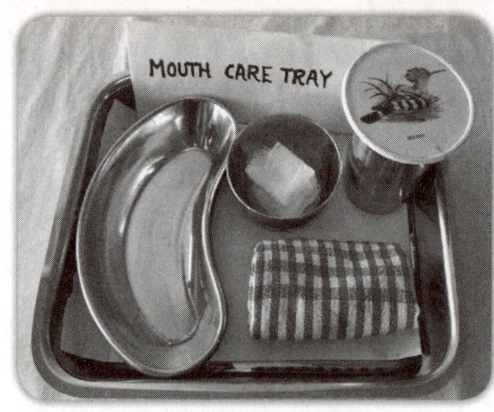

Fig. 19: A tray containing the articles for the mouth care

Procedure

Steps of Procedure	Rationale
• Wash hands properly	• To prevent infection
• Warp the gauze or cloth around the finger and damp it with water	• To clean the mouth easily
• Gently put the finger inside the baby's mouth	• To prevent friction

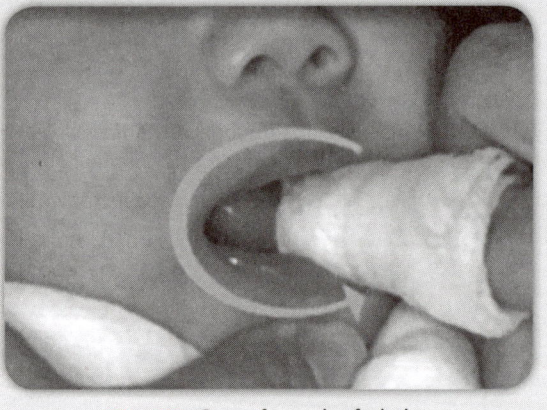

Figs 20: Care of mouth of a baby

• Wipe the upper and then lower gum pad once	• To remove milk stains and remove/reduce bad odor
• Discard the gauze	• Waste products
• Recording and reporting	• Report for redness or crack/cheilosis in mouth
• Give health education to mother	• To gain knowledge

Points to Remember

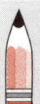

- Clean hands and the cloth to be used
- Do not clean the mouth immediately after breastfeeding, baby can vomit.

CARE OF BUTTOCKS

Purposes

- To prevent infection
- To prevent nappy rash
- To keep the area clean and dry.

Equipments Needed

A clean small tray containing the following articles (**Fig. 21**):

- A bowl of warm water
- Cotton swabs
- Kidney tray
- A pair of clothes
- Diaper and nappy

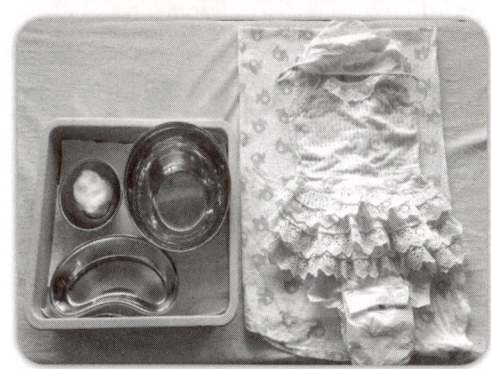

Fig. 21: A tray containing articles for the care of buttocks

Procedure

Steps of procedure	Rationale
• Wash the hands properly	• Prevent cross infection
• While cleaning the baby girl—wet a cotton ball, hold her legs apart and wipe between the labia with the cotton ball. Start at the front and gently wipe backward (**Fig. 22**).	• To prevent soiling

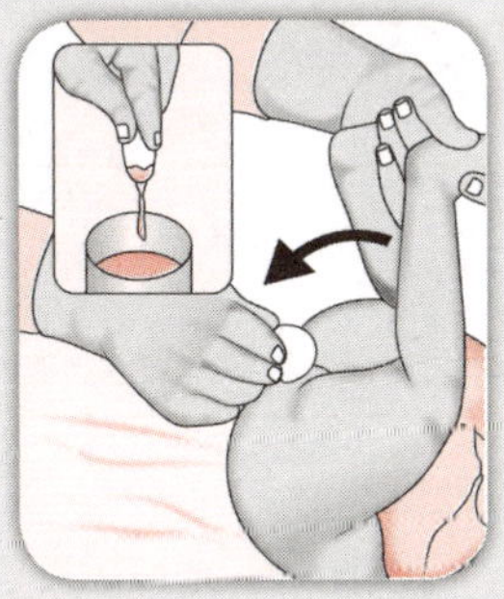

Fig. 22: Care of buttocks of a baby

• Dry it with a small towel	• To avoid moist and irritation
• For baby boys, gently rinse the genital area with water while cleaning (**Fig. 23**)	• To feel fresh and avoid infection

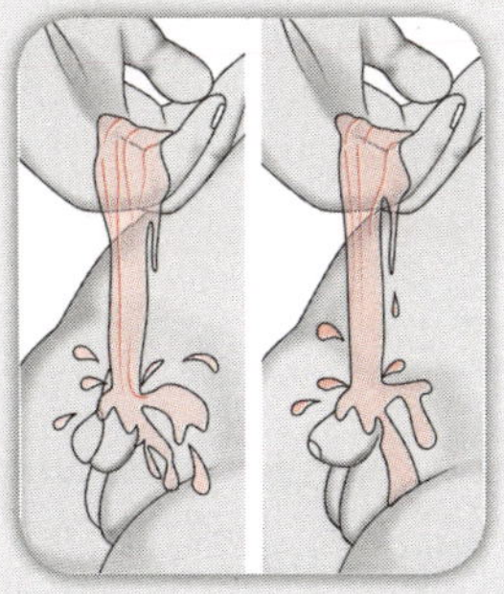

Fig. 23: Rinsing the genital area with water

Contd...

Steps of procedure	Rationale
• Wipe the back area with cotton balls	• To avoid friction
• Lastly wipe the anus area. Dry it with a small towel	• To avoid contamination
• Apply nappy ointment, if rash present. Put diaper and clothes	• To prevent rash
• Wash the hands	• To prevent cross infection
• Recording and reporting	
• Health education	• Gain knowledge
• Give your baby some 'nappy-free' time, and expose the skin **(Fig. 24)** 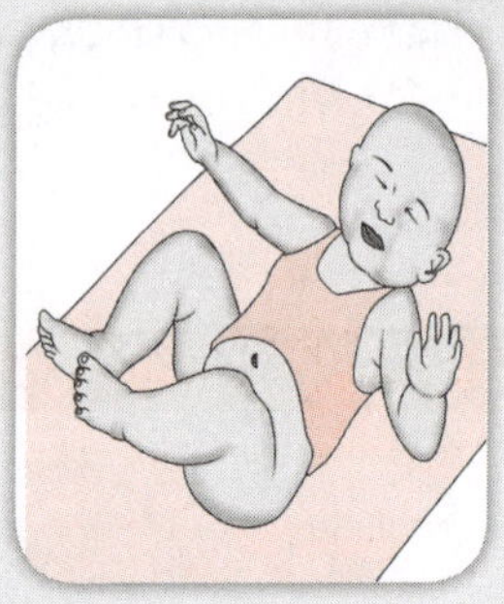	• For fast drying and healing • To prevent nappy rash.

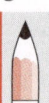

Fig. 24: Nappy free time to expose the skin and prevent infection and rash

Points to Remember

• Do not cover the umbilical cord
• Frequently change the diaper to avoid nappy rash.

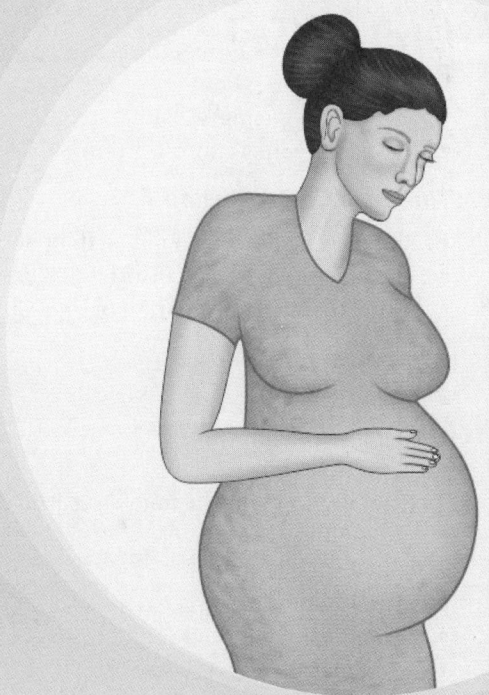

GYNECOLOGICAL PROCEDURES

ASSISTING WITH COPPER T INSERTION AND REMOVAL

Insertion of Cu-T

Purposes

- For birth spacing
- For emergency contraception.

Timing of Cu-T insertion

- Six weeks following child birth or abortion and 3 months after cesarean section
- Its preferable time to insert is 2–3 days after completion of menses
- After medical termination of pregnancy (MTP) and dilatation and curettage.

Equipments Needed

- Screen
- Draping sheet
- Mackintosh

A clean tray contains the following articles (**Fig. 1**):

- Vulsellum
- Sim's speculum
- Uterine sound
- Sponge holder
- Perineal sheet
- A pair of scissors
- A sterile Cu-T in a packet
- A pair of sterile gloves
- A bowl containing sterile savlon/dettol soaked swabs

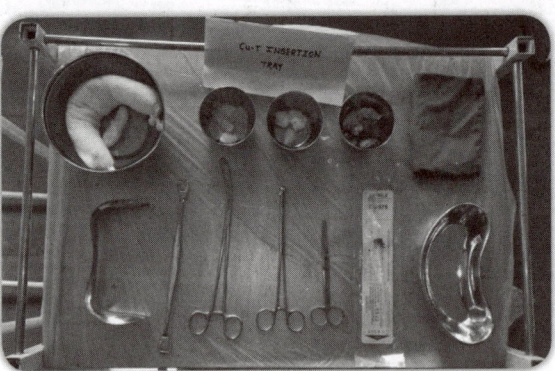

Fig. 1: A tray containing articles for Cu-T insertion

Procedure

Steps of procedure	Rationale
• Provide privacy	• To ensure safe and secure feel for patient
• Explain the procedure	• To reduce anxiety
• Wash hands and keep the articles near by	• To prevent cross infection

Contd...

Steps of procedure	Rationale
• Place the patient in dorsal position and clean the perineum	• To visualize the perineum and aseptic measures used
• Insert the vaginal speculum	• To inspect vagina
• Hold the anterior lip of the cervix with the help of Allis forceps and clean using antiseptic solution	• To prevent infection
• Pass the uterine sound through cervical canal	• To note the position of the uterus and the length of the uterine cavity
• Cu-T device is loaded	
• The inserter with the device placed inside then introduced through cervical canal right up to the fundus after positioning it by guard	• To avoid pulling the tail of the intrauterine contraceptive device (IUCD)
• The Allis forceps is handed over to assistant and the inserter with right hand withdrawn keeping the plunger in position and pushing the Cu-T out. **(Fig. 2)**	• To avoid discomfort and also helps to locate the IUCD in situ

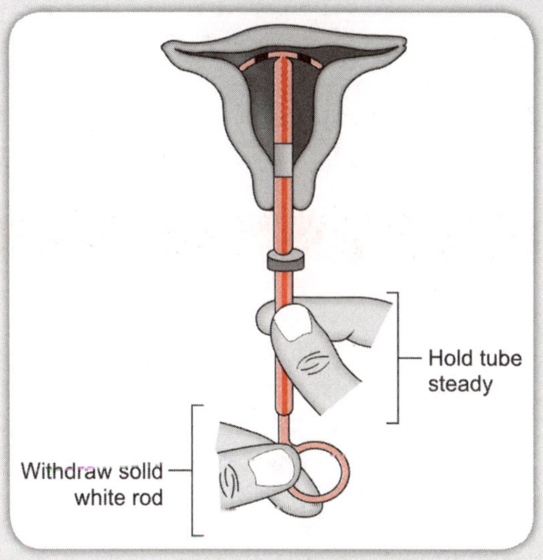

Fig. 2: Cu-T insertion

• The plunger is removed first, followed by the removal of the inserter.	
• The strings of the thread are cut from the external os and less thread is left out	
• Woman rests for 15–20 minutes and thereafter leaves	• To feel relaxed and comfort
• Record and report the findings	• To ensure SMART documentation

Removal of Cu-T

Removal of Cu-T may occur at any time in the menstrual cycle but it may be earliest during menses or mid-cycles.

Procedure

Steps of procedure	Rationale
• Patient is positioned as for the insertion of IUCD	• To inspect the vagina and cervix
• Wear sterile gloves	• To prevent cross infection
• Clean the vulva and vagina with 1% savlon and insert sterile speculum into the vagina, locate the thread	• To perform aspectic measures
• Apply steady gentle traction and pull the string with long artery forceps	• Pulling leads in removal of IUCD
• Ensure that Cu-T which is removed, checked and shown to the patient and discarded	• To avoid remaining of few parts of IUCD inside the uterus
• Recording and reporting and give health education	• To ensure SMART documentation and maintain hygiene

Points to Remember

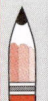

- To be inserted on the 5th or 6th day after menstruation
- Relax the perineal muscles
- Notify the doctor, if there is excessive pain, bleeding and any other discomforts.

ASSISTING WITH PAP SMEAR

Pap Smear Tests
- In this test, sample of exfoliated cell (dead cells that are shed) are obtained
- This specimen should be obtained 2 weeks after the first day of last menstrual period (LMP) by bruising or scraping.

Purpose
- To detect early cancer of the cervix
- To determine estrogen activity related to menopause abnormalities.

Equipments Needed
A clean tray containing the following articles (**Fig. 3**):
- Vaginal speculum
- Savlon solution and cotton swabs
- Perineal drapes
- Sterile gloves and mask
- Lubricant jelly
- Glass slide
- Torch light
- Cytobrush or swab sticks or Ayre's wooden spatula

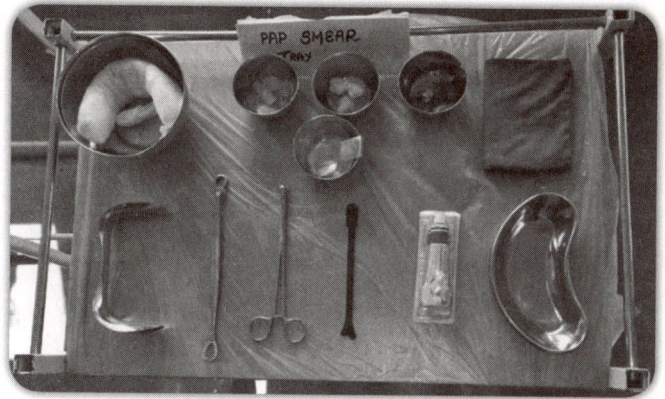

Fig. 3: A tray containing articles for pap smear test

Preliminary Assessment

- Explain the procedure to the patient (make sure that patient is not menstruating)
- Before appointment patient should avoid sexual intercourse, refrain from douching and cessation of vaginal medication for 2 days should be done
- Advice the patient to void and provide privacy

Procedure

Steps of procedure	Rationale
• Give dorsal position; drape the patient and during procedure, encourage the patients to take deep breaths	• To permit minimal exposure and to relax the abdominal muscles
• Insert the speculum	• To inspect the vagina and cervix
• Assist the physician **(Fig. 4)**	• To hold the speculum and torch light to focus the area

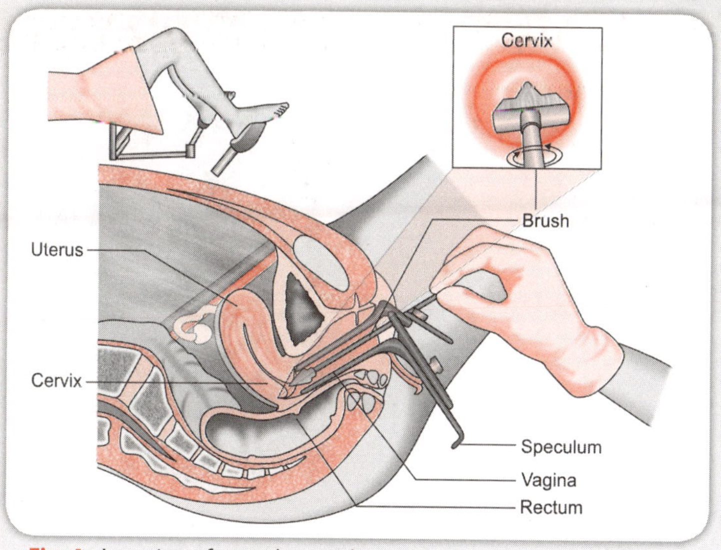

Cervix

Brush

Uterus

Cervix

Speculum

Vagina

Rectum

Fig. 4: Insertion of speculum and Visualization of Cervix and vagina

Contd...

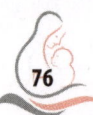
Steps of procedure	Rationale
• Use of cytobrush or with the help spatula rotate and scarps the cells and smeared onto glass slide, sprayed with a preservative to protect cells. **(Fig. 5)**	• To scrap the cells

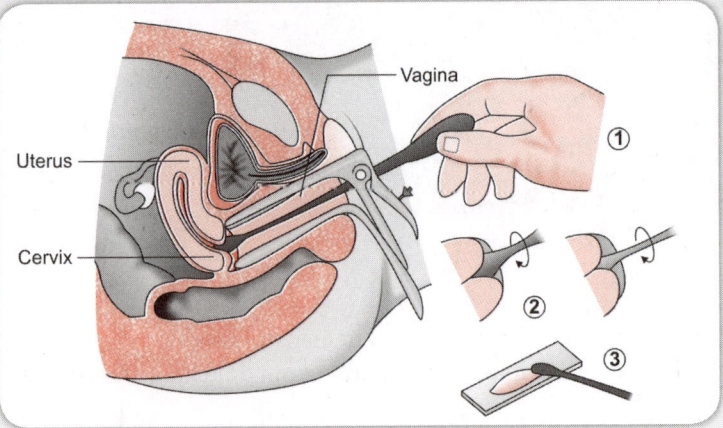

Fig. 5: Taking the sample of cells from the wall of cervix with help of cytobrush/spatula

Steps of procedure	Rationale
• Observe for any discharge, perineal care is done	• To avoid infection/menorrhagia
• Send the specimens to the laboratory	• To know status of cervical cancer
• Hand washing and replace the articles	
• Recording and reporting the abnormal findings and notify to the physician.	• To notify the doctor and give treatment as soon as possible

INSERTION OF PESSARY

Pessaries are medical devices inserted in the vagina.

Purposes
• To support the vaginal wall
• To correct the position or displace pelvic organs.

Equipments Needed
A clean tray containing the following articles:
• Sterile pack pessaries
• Vaginal speculum
• Antiseptic solution
• Lubricant jelly

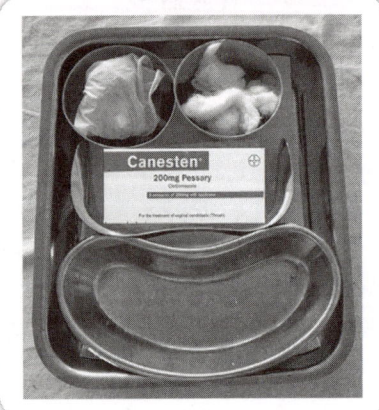

Procedure

Steps of procedure	Rationale
• Explain the procedure to the patient	• To get cooperation
• Provide privacy	• To limit exposure
• Wash the hands properly	• To prevent cross infection
• Give dorsal position and clean the perineal area with antiseptic solution	• Easy visualization
• Remove the pessary from the sterile pack	• To use aseptic measures
• Note the size of the pessaries according the size of vagina and cervix	• To fit inside
• Grab the pessary and fold in half	• For easy insertion
• Apply lubricant to the pessary (note the curved position should be faced upward, toward the ceiling as you hold the pessary)	• To avoid contamination
• Position the patient and spread the labia with nondominant hand, fold the pessary in dominant hand	• To avoid discomfort
• Carefully push the folded lubricated pessary into the vagina, push it back as far as possible without causing discomfort **(Fig. 6)**	• Prevent cross infection

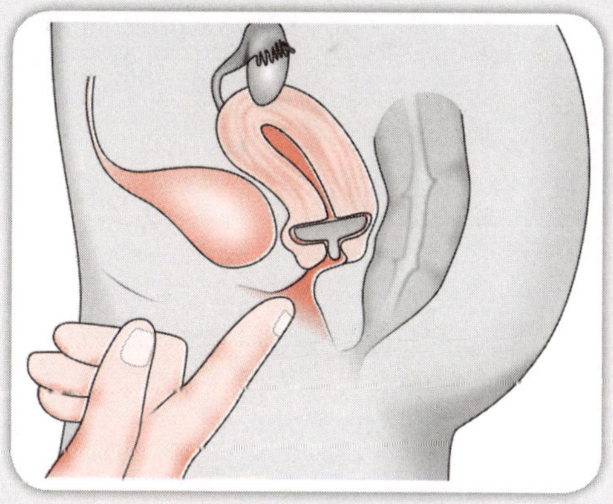

Fig. 6: Insertion of pessary

• Release the pessary (it will unfold and return to its normal shape)	
• Hand washing and replace the articles	
• Recording and reporting	• Ensure SMART documentation
• Health education	

Point to Remember

• Removal is done same as after every 15 days and maintain personal hygiene to prevent the infection.

NONAPPLICATOR TAMPON INSERTION

Purpose

To avoid excessive menstrual bleeding

Equipments Needed

A clean tray containing the following articles (**Fig. 7**)

- Tampon
- Gloves
- Lubricant jelly, if required.

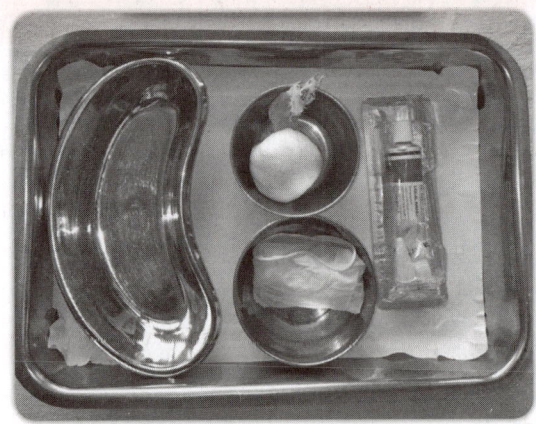

Fig. 7: A tray containing articles for nonapplicator tampon insertion

Procedure

Steps of procedure	Rationale
• Wash the hands with soap and water	• To prevent infection
• With dry hands, unwrap the tampon (**Fig. 8**)	• To avoid as much contact with the tampon as possible to prevent infection

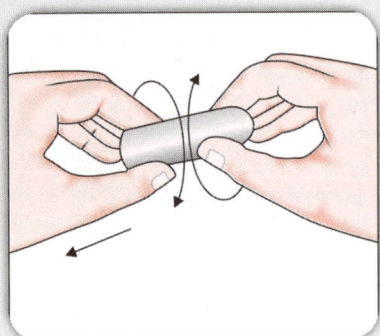

Fig. 8: Unwrapping the tampon

• Holding the part of the tampon that is still wrapped pull out the string, ensuring that it is securely attached to the tampon. **(Figs 9A to C)**

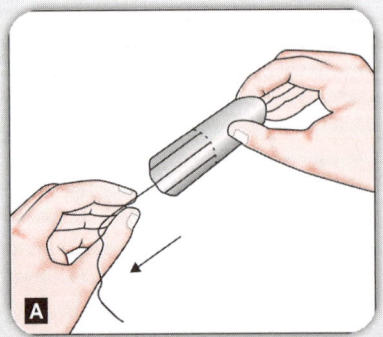

Contd...

Steps of procedure	Rationale

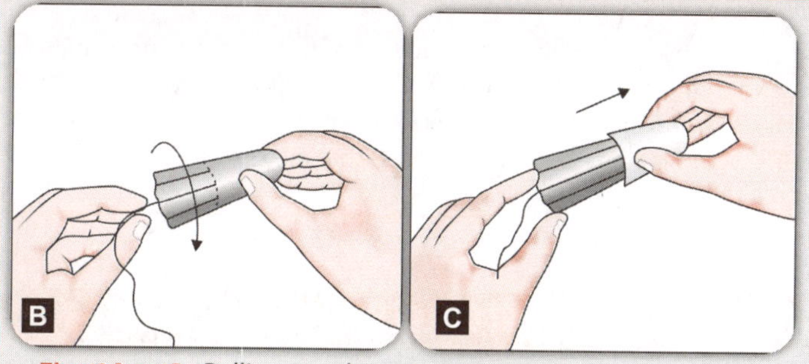

Figs 9A to C: Pulling out-the string to ensure that it is properly attached to the tampon

Steps of procedure	Rationale
• Sit or stand in a comfortable position. Some women prefer to place one leg up on the toilet seat, while others prefer to sit down on the toilet with their legs slightly apart. It is entirely up to patients comfort	• To be in comfortable position for easy insertion
• Relax and then push the tampon into the vagina **(Fig. 10)**	• For easy insertion

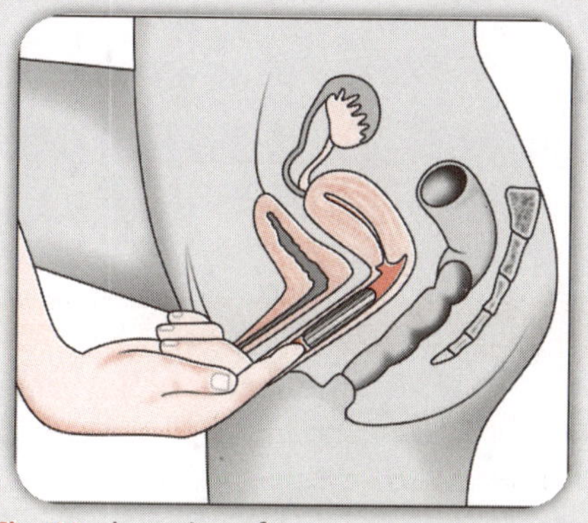

Fig. 10: Insertion of tampon into the vagina

Steps of procedure	Rationale
• The string should hang down so that it can be pulled on it when want to remove it. **(Fig. 11)**	• Helps in pulling down the tampon

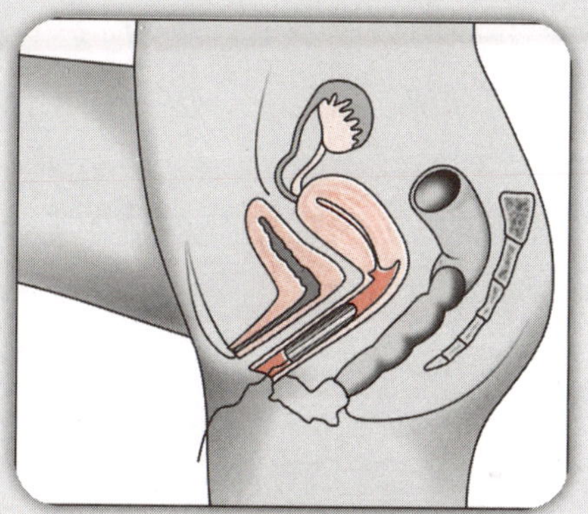

Fig. 11: Inserting tampon in such a way so that string should hang down

Steps of procedure	Rationale
• Wash the hands again; dispose the wrapper in a bin.	• To prevent cross infection

Points to Remember

- The tampon can be removed slowly by pulling the string downward and forward. Once the tampon has been removed, wrap in the toilet tissue and throw away in the waste bin.
- Always use the correct absorbency for the flow and change the tampon every 4 to 6 hours. Tampons are associated with toxic shock syndrome (TSS). This is a rare but serious illness that may be fatal.

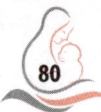

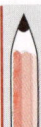

INSERTION OF SUPPOSITORIES

Suppositories are in different shapes and it will get melted/dissolved according to a body temperature. Two types of suppositories are available—rectal and vaginal.

Rectal Suppositories

Purposes

- To treat infection
- For medication purpose.

Equipments Needed

- Suppositories
- Gloves.

Procedure

Steps of procedure	Rationale
Rectal suppositories • Explain the procedure to the patient	• To get cooperation
• Encourage the patient to void and give privacy	• To ensure wellbeing
• Remove the wrapper	• To insert
• Moisten the suppository with water or lubricant jelly	• For easy insertion
• Advice the patient to lie on left side	• To get proper anatomical position
• Gently push the suppositories into the rectum, so it is deep enough not to come out **(Fig. 12)** **Fig. 12:** Insertion of rectal suppositories	• To avoid spilling out

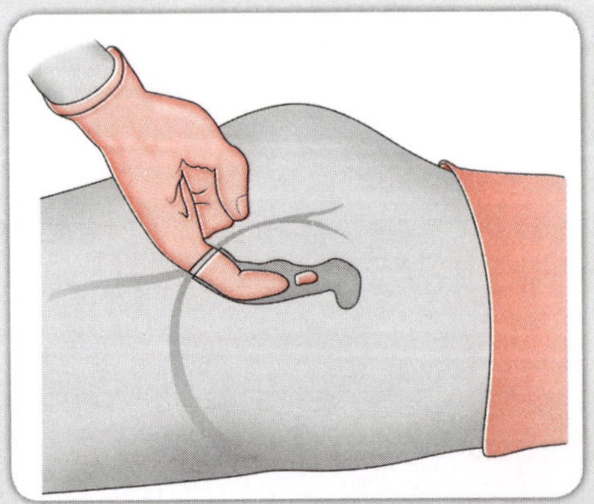

Contd...

Steps of procedure	Rationale
• Wash the hands properly	• To prevent cross infection
• Recording and reporting	• To ensure SMART documentation
• Health education	• To gain knowledge

Vaginal Suppositores/Tablets/Creams

Purpose

- To treat gynecological ailments (candidiasis)
- Best time to insert these products at bed time.

Procedure

Steps of procedure	Rationale
• Clean the perineal area and dry it	• To avoid infection
• For **vaginal cream products**: Attach the applicators to the opening of the tube cream and twist until firmly attached	• To insert inside the vagina
• Squeeze the cream from the tube into the applicator (required dose)	• Do not waste the cream
• For **suppositories**: Unwrap the suppositories and place into the end of the applicator	• Helps in easy insertion
• Gently insert the applicator into the vagina in a standing or lying position (knee bent and legs slightly apart) **(Fig. 13)**	• Proper position for easy insertion

Fig. 13: Insertion of vaginal suppositories

• Push the plunger of the applicator until it reaches the top. Remove the applicator from the vagina	
• Hand washing and recording and reporting	• Prevent cross infection and SMART documentation
• Continue the use of medication for as long as directed by the doctor	• For further treatment

Points to Remember

- Maintain personal hygiene
- Notify the doctors for any signs of infection

NOTE

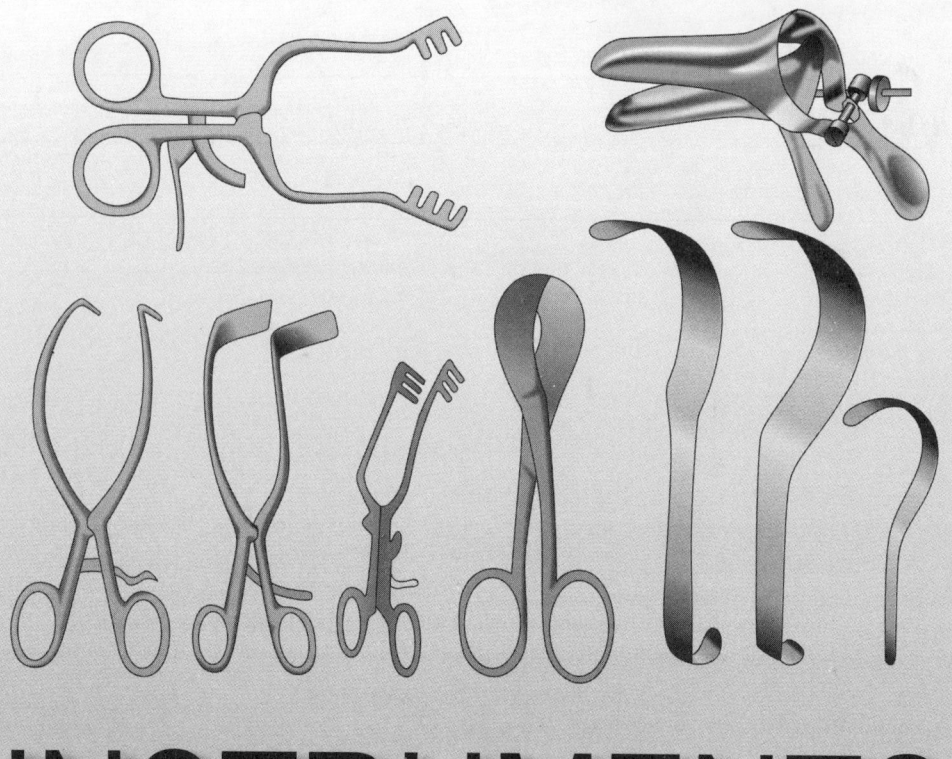

INSTRUMENTS

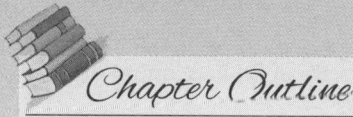

Chapter Outline

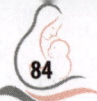

SPECULUM

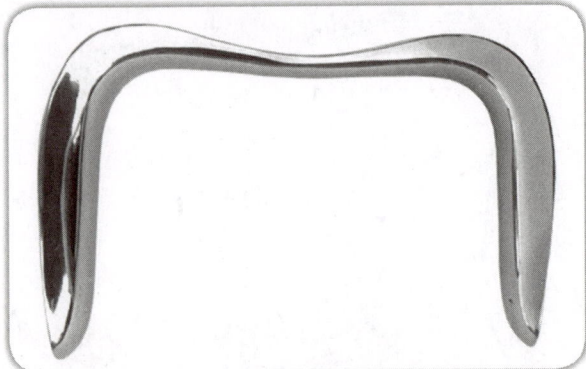

Fig. 1: Sim's speculum

A vaginal speculum is an instrument which allows inspection of the vagina by retracting vaginal walls. Speculums are made of stainless steel and are sterilized by boiling or autoclaving.

SIMS' Speculum (Duck-Bill Speculum) (Fig. 1)

Features
- Speculum are made of stainless steel.
- Either double ended or single ended.
- If double ended, each end is of different sizes (26 and 31 mm, 31 and 36 mm, 36 and 41 mm).
- Blades are rounded and a traumatic.
- Broad end is used for multipara and thin end is used for primipara.

Uses
- Used to retract the vaginal wall, usually the posterior wall to inspect.
- To examine cervix and vagina for discharge, cervicitis, polyps, prolapse, carcinoma and malformations.
- To carry out biopsy, dilatation and curettage, hystero salpin gogram, hysteroscopy, vaginal hysterectomies, colpotomy/culdocentesis.
- To examine cervical or vaginal tears.
- Endometrial biopsy or cervical biopsy.
- Insertion or removal of an intrauterine contraceptive device (IUCD).
- The handle is slightly concave to collect drained blood and secretions.
- To pack the uterine cavity in atonic postpartum hemorrhage.

Directions to Use
- Patient needs to be at the edge of the table and in dorsal position.
- Speculum is lubricated with antiseptic solution or jelly.
- Labia minora are held apart by thumb and index finger of the left hand and blade inserted with its transverse axis along the long axis of the labia.
- Blade is rotated in vagina by 90° to retract the posterior wall of the vagina.
- Posterior wall is examined as the blade is withdrawn.
- Anterior vaginal wall retractor is used along with Sims' speculum for better visualization.

Cusco Speculum (Fig. 2)

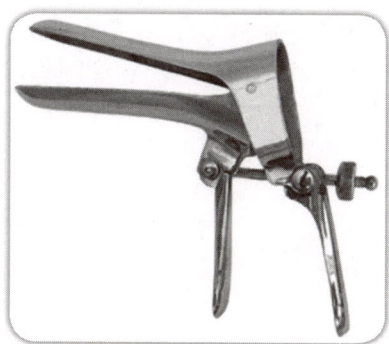

Fig. 2: Cusco speculum

Features

- It has two blades connected by a hinge so they open and close around transverse axis.
- Concave inside and round ends.
- It can be used in vagina in different sizes.
- Upper blade has a notch at its outer end, through which vulsellum may be passed inside without obstructing the field of vision.

Uses

- Inspection of the vagina and the cervix as Sims' speculum.
- It is a self-retaining speculum, it dispense with the need for an assistant to hold it.
- Cervical biopsy, insertion of IUCD.
- To perform pap smear.
- It cannot be used for procedures because it covers the anterior and posterior vaginal wall.

Directions to Use

- The lubricated closed blades are passed between labia minora, transverse axis of the blades in the long axis of the labia.
- Once inside the vagina the blades are rotated to 90° and are opened till the cervix is exposed satisfactorily.
- The blades are fixed in this position by the butterfly screw.

ANTERIOR VAGINAL WALL RETRACTOR (Fig. 3)

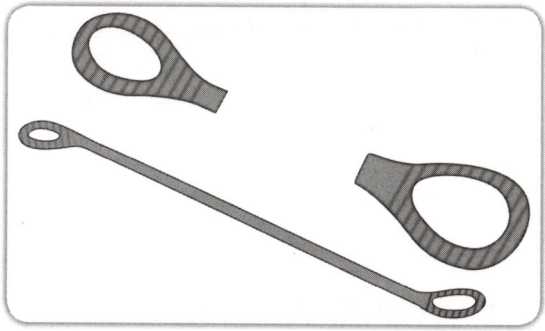

Fig. 3: Anterior vaginal wall retractor

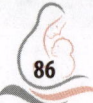

Features

- Long instrument with spoon shaped ends which have transverse serrations on either surface.
- The loops make an angle of 15° with the shaft and are angled in opposite directions.

Uses

- Retraction of the anterior vaginal wall to expose the cervix in conjunction with Sims' speculum.
- Used in cystocele.
- Blunt curettage.

Directions to Use

- Anterior vaginal wall retractor used in conjunction with Sims' speculum during exposure of cervix. The transverse serrations on its looped ends provide friction against rugous vaginal mucosa and aid in efficient retraction.
- It is used as curettage after delivery or in mid trimester abortion.

EPISIOTOMY SCISSORS (Fig. 4)

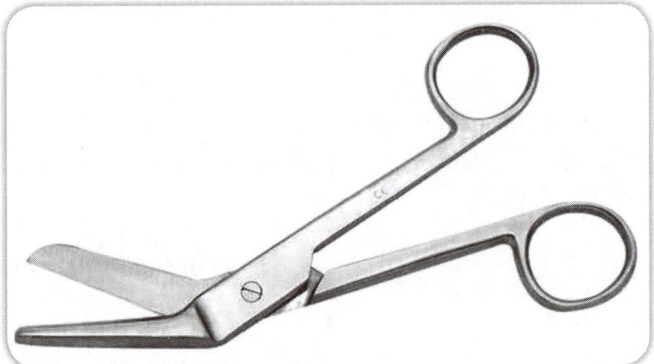

Fig. 4: Episiotomy scissors

Features

- Episiotomy scissors are 16 cm long.
- The blades are angled on the side. One side is sharp end and other end is blunt.

Uses

- To cut or widen the perineum in the following order:
  - Posterior vaginal wall, superficial and deep transverse perineal muscles.
  - Bulbospongiosus, fascia covering the muscles.
  - Transverse perineal branch of pudendal vessels and nerves.
  - To avoid rectal tear and ease delivery of baby head.

Directions to Use

- The sharp blade of the instrument is inserted in the vagina protecting fetus by two fingers of the doctor.

- Shape allows easy introduction into the vagina and prevents erratic cutting.
- Angle prevents butting of the instrument against the patient's buttocks.
- The episiotomy is sutured in 3 layers with no 0 (one zero) chromic catgut. The first layer is vagina starting with the apex. The second layer is perineal muscles and the third layer is skin.
- The episiotomy can extend if proper perineal support is not given. Extension to anus is seen in median episiotomy.

TOWEL CLIP (Fig. 5)

Features

- Made up of stainless steel.
- Distal end has c shaped curvature.
- Has catch –lock mechanism.
- Available in different sizes.

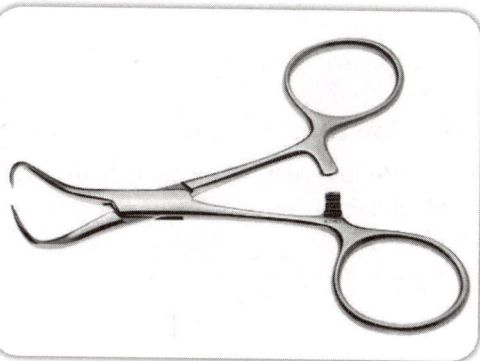

Uses

- It is used in draping the operative area abdominal or vaginal.
- The towels or sheets are fixed to the skin and each other with these clips.
- Used during lower segment cesarean section (LSCS).

Fig. 5: Towel clip

Direction to Use

- Distal end used to fix up drape and instrument can be locked.

BLAKE'S UTERINE CURRETTE (Fig. 6)

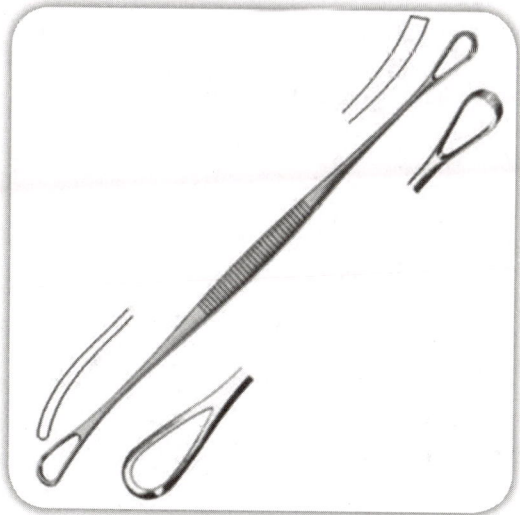

Fig. 6: Blake's uterine currette

Features

- It has central shaft and one small oval loop at each end.
- The two loops are angles in opposite directions.
- The size of the loops varies from 2 × 3 mm to 6 × 10 mm.
- The edge of the loop is either sharp or blunt.

Uses

- To take an endometrial sample in cases of abnormal vaginal bleeding.
- To detect ovulation in cases of infertility by detection of secretory change of endometrium.
- To remove the decidua (curette) after evacuation in case of abortion and molar pregnancy.
- To remove retained products of conception in cases of postpartum hemorrhage.

Direction to Use

- The loops are set at an angle to the shaft so that tip of the loop is directed away from the direction of the shaft and can curette the endometrium easily.

PLACENTA CURETTE (Fig. 7)

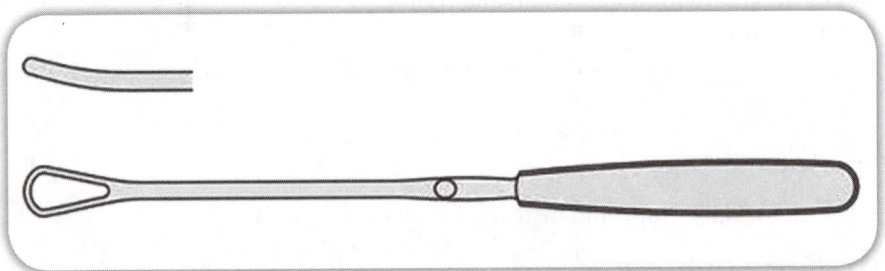

Fig. 7: Placenta curette

Features

- It has wide looped end for curetting and a handle at the other end.
- The edges of the loop are blunt.

Uses

- Check through curettage for incomplete abortion and retention of the placenta in second trimester abortions and retained segments or bits of placenta after delivery of a viable fetus.

Directions to Use

- The curette is introduced into uterine cavity after dilatation of cervix up to fundus and is withdrawn, its sharp curetting edge scraping against the endometrium.
- All the walls of the uterine cavity are systematically curetted.

SIMPSON'S UTERINE SOUND (Fig. 8)

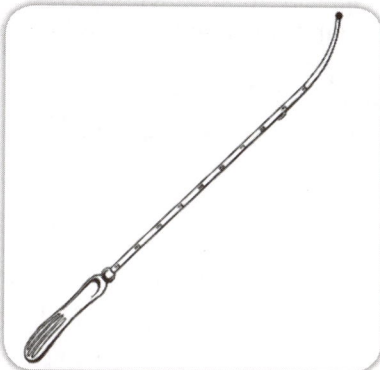

Fig. 8: Simpson's uterine sound

Features

- It is 30 cm long, of which 5 cm length is that of its handle.
- Rest of the instrument is graduated in inches or centimeter.
- It bends at an angle of 150° at a distance of 2.5 inches from its tip at a distance of normal uterocervical length.
- The sound is olive tipped.

Uses

- To measure the length of the uterine cavity.
- To know the position and direction of the uterus in case of retroversion.
- To differentiate between a polyp arising from the cervical canal or body of the uterus.
- To measure the length of the cervical canal.

Direction to Use

- Instrument use by exerting pressure from wrist joint only
- Be gentle during use.
- Curvature to be used as per position of uterus (anteverted or retroverted)

DITTEL BLADDER SOUND (Fig. 9)

Features

- It is usually 25 cm long.
- It has a handle and a long rod shaped sounding portion which is curved in its terminal 5 cm.
- It is available in different sizes.
- The bladder sounds differ from uterine sound in that it has no angulations but a smooth curve and it's not graduated.
- It does not have a tip like uterine sound.

Fig. 9: Dittel bladder sound

Uses

- Diagnosis of accidental bladder injury during obstetrics or gynecological operations.
- To define the limit of the bladder during operations on the anterior vaginal wall to safeguard it form injury.
- To define the position of a vesicovaginal fistula opening in the vagina.
- To sound the urinary bladder for foreign body, e.g. stone, perforated intrauterine contraceptive device (IUCD).

Directions to Use

- The bladder sound is passed through urethra into the bladder and its tips are maneuvered till they emerge through the dent in the bladder wall.

BABCOCKS FORCEPS (Fig. 10)

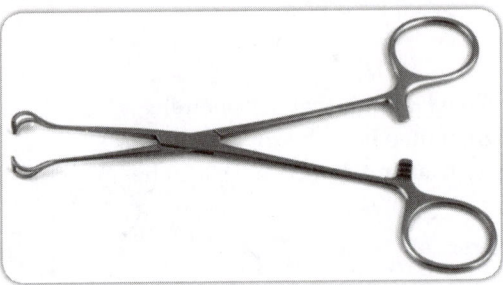

Fig. 10: Babcocks forceps

Features

- This instrument has fenestrated triangular blades and grooved jaws.
- It is available in three sizes: large, medium and small.
- The large and medium sized forceps have identical blades and they differ in their lengths like 12 and 17 respectively.
- The small forceps is 10 cm long and has small blades.
- It is nontraumatic instruments.

Uses

- To hold the Fallopian tubes in the following operations like tubal ligation, tuboplasty and salpingectomy.
- To hold bladder during repair of accidental injury to the bladder and vesicovaginal fistula repair.
- To hold uterus in ovarian tumors and dissection of ureter.
- To hold ovary in ovarian cystectomy etc.

Direction to Use

- Fallopian tubes to be catch properly in between grooved jaws of the instrument avoid any injury to tubular structure.
- During tubectomy use two Babcocks frorceps to catch fallopian tube and cut and ligate in between two babcocks.

CERIVAL DILATORS (HEGARS/FENTONS DILATORS) (Fig. 11)

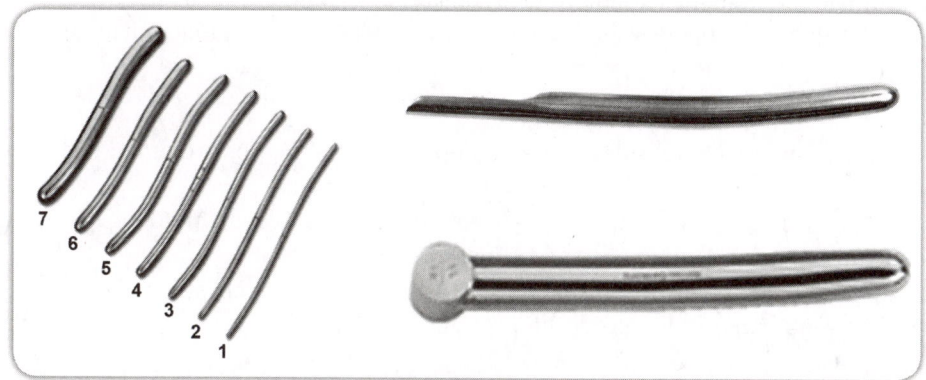

Fig. 11: Cerival dilators

Features

- This instrument may be single ended or double ended.
- It is a solid rod curve near the top and somewhat tapering toward the tip.
- The curve is shallow and the dilating portion is within terminal 1.5 cm of the dilator.
- These dilators are numbered from 3/6 to 23/26.

Uses

- Prior to endometrial curettage.
- Prior to suction aspiration for first trimester pregnancy termination.
- Prior to suction evacuation of a vesicular mole is done.
- Removal of endometrial polyps.
- Removal of IUCD, hysteroscopy and cervical stenosis.

Direction to Use

- Use instrument in pen fashion.
- Exert pressure only from wrist.
- Remember instrument only for dilating stenosed cervix, so avoid deeper insertion to prevent uterine perforation.
- Maximum size to be used is No 2 more than that of weeks of gestation.

GREEN ARMYTAGE FORCEPS (Fig. 12)

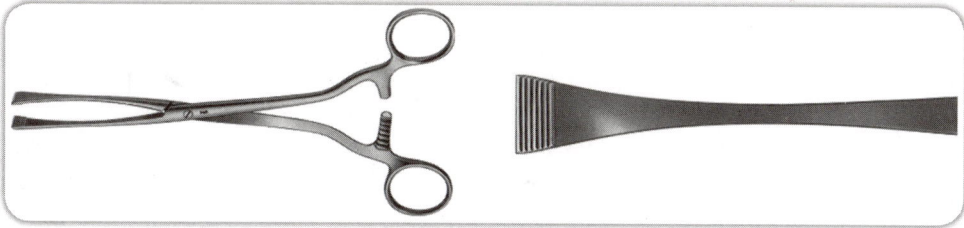

Fig. 12: Green armytage forceps

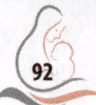
Features

- This instrument has triangular solid tips with transverse serrations.
- A ratchet lock makes its grip secure.

Uses

- This forceps is used as a hemostat in cesarean operation. As the tips are broad wide area can be compressed.
- In lower segment cesarean section (LSCS) the cut uterine edges bleed, this forceps is applied to the two angles and lower and upper edge of the incision.
- The common indications for LSCS are fetal distress in first stage, chronic pelvic disease (CPD), abnormal presentations like transverse lie, brow, breech in primi, previous two scars on the uterus.

Direction to Use

- As it has broader wide tip it catches more surface during hemostasis.
- Catch wide active bleeder and lock forceps.
- Multiple forceps can be used for more effective result.

NEEDLE HOLDER (Fig. 13)

Features

- The inner surface of tip has serrations and a small grove for firm grasp of the curved needle.
- The box joint is placed very close to tip to give adequate pressure because of the lever effect.
- Available in different sizes

Uses

This instrument is used for grasping needle at the time of suturing.

Direction to Use

- Use small or large size of needle holder as per convenience.
- Needle to be hold in such fashion that holder divides needle anterior 2/3rd and posterior 1/3rd
- Before using make sure effective locking system of instrument.

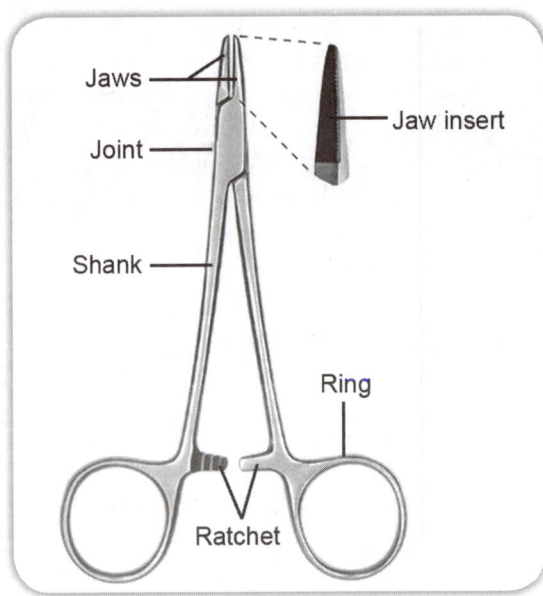

Fig. 13: Needle holder

OVUM FORCEPS (Fig. 14)

Features

- This instrument is a nonlocking forceps and has spoon-shaped ends.
- It has hinged at one ends and some of which may be hinged only in center.
- The forceps allows the objects to be grasped easily in a closed position so that they can be manipulated and stay in place while the procedure is being performed.

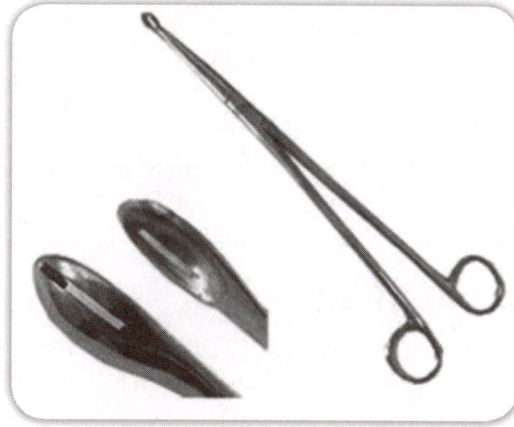

Fig. 14: Ovum forceps

Uses

- This instrument is used for removing the products of conception is inevitable, incomplete abortion and in medical termination of pregnancy (MTP) operations.
- The tip of this instrument is rounded cup like to avoid perforation and to hold large tissue.
- This instrument has no catch. This is to avoid perforation of wall.

Direction to Use

- Exert pressure only from wrist.
- Remember instrument to be used after dilating stenosed cervix.
- While introducing and removing instrument from cervical canal, always close spoon shaped ends.
- Remove product of conception in twisted manner.

KOCHER'S FORCEPS (Fig. 15)

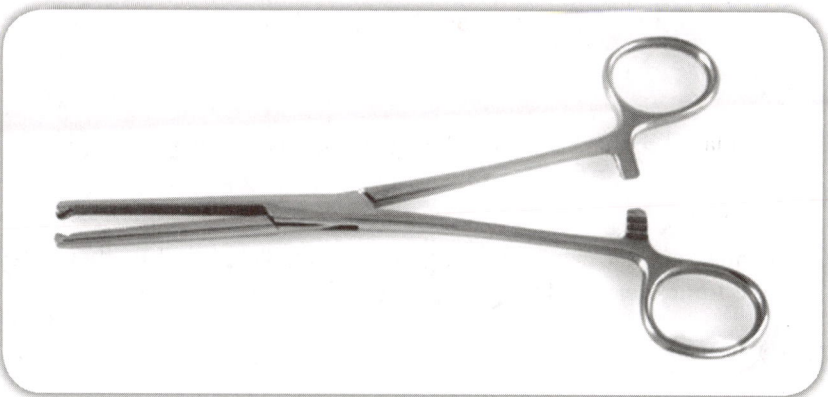

Fig. 15: Kocher's forceps

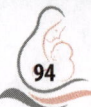

Features

- Strong straight metal instruments.
- Has a catch lock to bring the blades together for locking.
- Inner surface of the both blades are transversely serrated.
- Single tooth at distal end.

Uses

- To catch the edges of the incision, while suturing skin.
- Used for artificial rupture of membranes.
- Used to clamp the umbilical cord.

Direction to Use

- Confirm presence of bag of membrane while artificially rupturing.
- Depressed part of presentation by index and middle finger and rupture membrane in between.

AYRE'S SPATULA (Fig. 16)

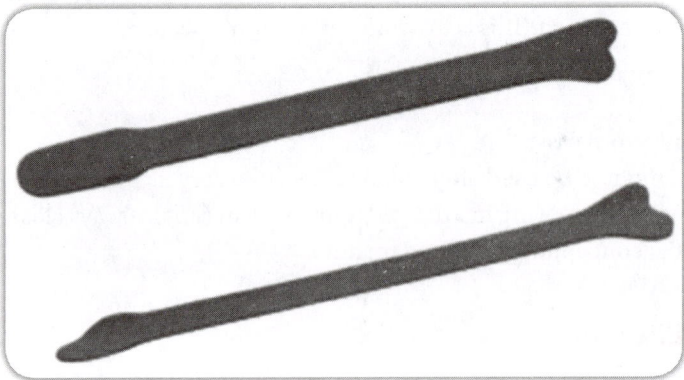

Fig. 16: Ayre's spatula

Feature

- Made of wood or plastic so that cells can adhere to its porous surface.

Uses

- It is used for taking Pap smear for screening of carcinoma cervix. The other broad end is used for obtaining cells from lateral vagina for knowing the hormonal status.

Directions to Use

- Lithotomy position is given, cervix is exposed with Sims' speculum and anterior vaginal wall retractor.
- The long end is inserted into cervical canal and rotated at 360°.
- The exfoliated cells obtained are smeared on glass slide and fixed in Koplicks jar which contains ether and alcohol in equal amount.

OBSTETRICAL FORCEPS (Fig. 17)

Feature

Obstetrical forceps are made up of stainless steel. Each forceps has two branches. Each branch has a blade with cephalic and pelvic curves, a handle and a shank. Two branches connected by a lock.

Uses

- During forceps delivery.
- To delivered after coming head in breech delivery.

Directions to Use

- Lithotomy position given to mother.
- Bladder catheterized and emptied.
- Vaginal examination done to see prerequisites have been satisfied.
- Episiotomy given.
- Checked forceps for correct pair.
- Outer surface of blade is lubricated. Left and right blades are inserted respectively.
- Locked forceps.
- Forward and upward traction are given during uterine contractions.
- Forceps is unlocked and removed as soon as head delivers.

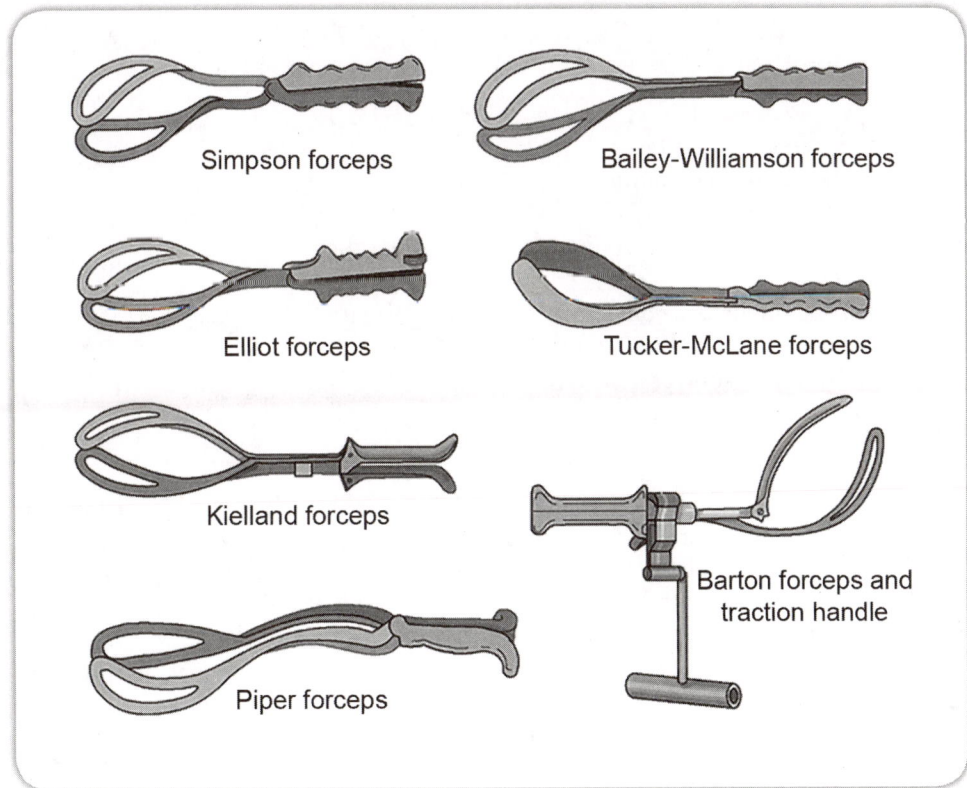

Simpson forceps

Bailey-Williamson forceps

Elliot forceps

Tucker-McLane forceps

Kielland forceps

Barton forceps and traction handle

Piper forceps

Fig. 17: Types of obstetrical forceps

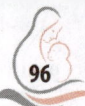
VACUUM EXTRACTOR (Fig. 18)

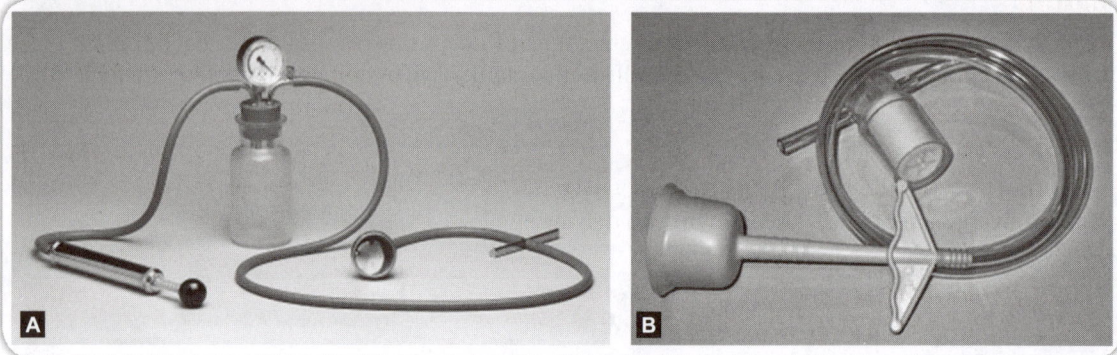

Fig. 18: Vacuum extractor

Features

A vacuum extractor has a suction cup, a traction handle, a source of creating vacuum and vacuum gauge to note the negative pressure created. The cup may be made of metal or silicone material. The source of vacuum may be hand operated pump, or an electric pump. The cup is available in 4 sizes 30, 40, 50 and 60 mm in diameter. The depth of cup is 20 mm.

Use

During vacuum delivery.

Directions to Use

- Lithotomy position is given to mother.
- Bladder is catheterized and emptied.
- Vaginal examination done to see prerequisites have been satisfied.
- Episiotomy is given.
- Cup is inserted and put in firm contact with fetal head. Vacuum of 0.8 kg/cm^2 is maintained.
- Perpendicular traction is made during uterine contractions.
- The vacuum is broken as soon as head delivers.

FETOSCOPE (Fig. 19)

Features

This instrument is made of either wood or aluminium. It is funnel shaped and has a broad flat disk with a central perforation attached at the narrow end of the funnel at right angle to the long axis of the funnel. The rim of the broad end is rounded to avoid pain to the patient by the edge cutting into the abdominal wall.

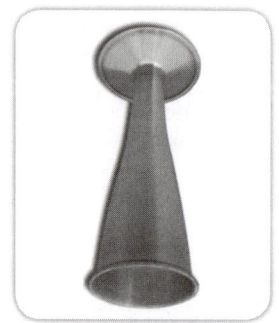

Use

For auscultation of fetal heart sound.

Fig. 19: Fetoscope

Directions to Use

- Warm the instrument at abdominal part to reduce fetal stimuli.
- Create vacuum for clarity of FHS.
- Do not touch instrument by hand while in use.
- Place patient in supine position with a lateral tilt of 15°. The position of anterior shoulder of fetus is determined and FHS best heard at this point except face presentation.

DOYEN'S RETRACTOR (Fig. 20)

Features

This instrument has curved sturdy blade and stout handle. Also a hole at middle of handle for easy grip during retraction.

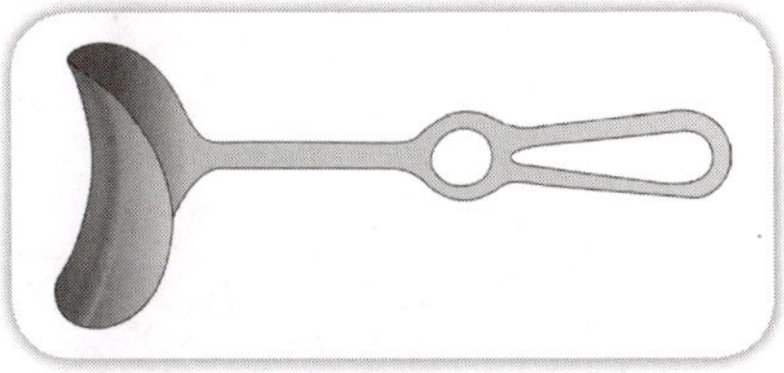

Uses

This instrument is used for retraction of the abdominal wall suprapubically during abdominal operations such as—

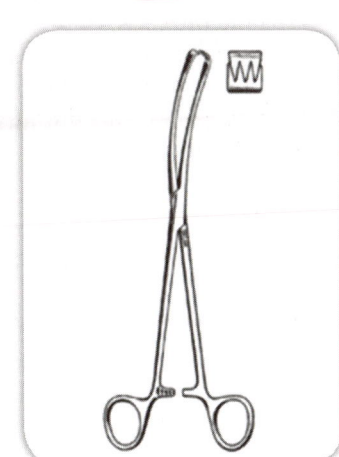

Fig. 20: Doyen's retractor

- Cesarean section.
- Operation for ruptured ectopic gestation.
- Obstetrical hysterectomies.
- Abdominal hysterectomies.
- Ovarian cystectomy, oophorectomy and wedge resection.
- Prolapsed repair surgeries.
- Stress urinary incontinence repair.

Directions to Use

This retractor is used after the peritoneum has been opened. The broad retracting surface achieves good retraction. The solid blade compresses the cut edges of the abdominal wall and achieves a hemostatic effect.

VULSELLUM (Fig. 21)

Features

This instrument is 28 cm long. Its blades are curved on side in a gentle manner. The tips of the blade have 2 in 3 teeth. These teeth give a good grip to structure held. The gentle curve in the blades ensures that the fingers do not obstruct the field of vision when the cervix is held during vaginal surgeries.

Uses

- To hold and steady the cervix.
- To hold uterine fundus during abdominal hysterectomy.
- To hold uterine fundus during vaginal hysterectomy.
- To hold a leiomyomatous polyp and twist it during vaginal myomectomy.

Fig. 21: Vulsellum

Directions to Use

- The gentle curve in the blades ensures that the fingers do not obstruct the field of vision when the cervix is held during vaginal surgeries.
- It is used in conjunction with Sims' speculum and anterior vaginal wall retractor.

ALLIS FORCEPS (Fig. 22)

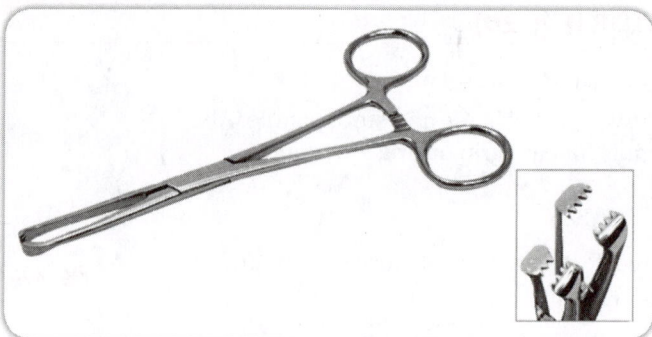

Fig. 22: Allis forceps

Features

This instrument is available in two sizes – 12 and 17 cm in length. Its blades are curved inward and have 4 in 5 or 5 in 6 teeth. A ratchet lock is present on the handles.

Uses

- To hold the cut edges of vagina in:
  - Abdominal hysterectomy.
  - Vaginal hysterectomy.
  - Anterior/posterior colporrhaphy.
  - Excision of vaginal wall cyst.
  - Enterocele repair.
  - Abdomino-peritoneal radical hysterectomy.
- To hold the cervix.
- To hold cut edges of rectus sheath.
- To hold cut edges of the lower segment for hemostasis as well as to aid its suturing in LSCS.
- To hold leiomyoma during myomectomy.
- To hold uterine fundus in vaginal and abdominal hysterectomy.

Direction to Use

- Catch tissue in between toothed area of forceps and lock it.

CORD CLAMP (Fig. 23)

Feature

Umbilical cord clamp is made of plastic to clamp a cord. It is disposable.

Use

- To clamp umbilical cord.

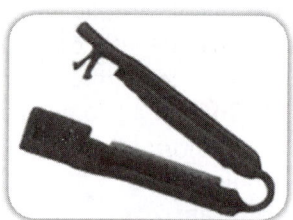

Fig. 23: Cord clamp

Direction to Use

- After receiving baby in baby unit, leaving 1–1$^1/_2$ cm cord stump this plastic cord clamp is applied and cord is cut above the clamp (site away from baby).

MUCUS SUCKER (Fig. 24)

Features

Mucus sucker is made of plastic, disposable instrument used for sucking mucus after birth. It has a suction tube, a tube for sucking and vacuum based specimen collection bottle.

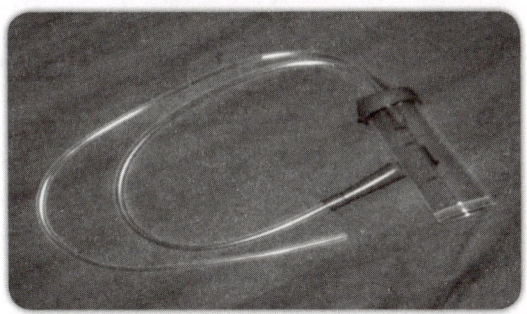

Uses

- For the suction of oronasal secretions.
- To send collected secretions for diagnostics.

Fig. 24: Mucus sucker

Directions to Use

- Suction tube to be inserted in baby's oral or nasal cavity.
- Sucking tube held in mouth and sucked.
- If vacuum machine is available it is attached to machine.
- Suctioning done and if required specimen bottle detached, covered, label and send to lab for diagnostics.

SHIRODKAR FORCEPS (Fig. 25)

Features

This is a long instrument made of stainless steel having a dome-shaped cavity to hold uterus. Blades have curved transverse bars at tip with distance in-between. Transverse bars have a gap to make it a traumatic.

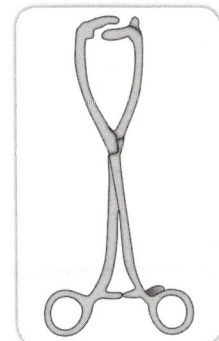

Use

- To hold and steady the uterus during operations.

Directions to Use

- Blades covered with rubber caps.
- Transverse bars have a gap to make it a traumatic.
- Bars occlude the isthmic region and cervical canal.
- Firm grip allows manipulation of uterus.

Fig. 25: Shirodkar forceps

BONNEY'S MYOMECTOMY CLAMP (Fig. 26)

Features

This is a long instrument with two pairs of finger grips, proximal and distal, with a ratchet lock on the handle near the proximal finger grips. The blades are at an angle of about 120° with the handles. The blades are covered with rubber caps distal to the site of the transverse bars.

Use

- During myomectomy.

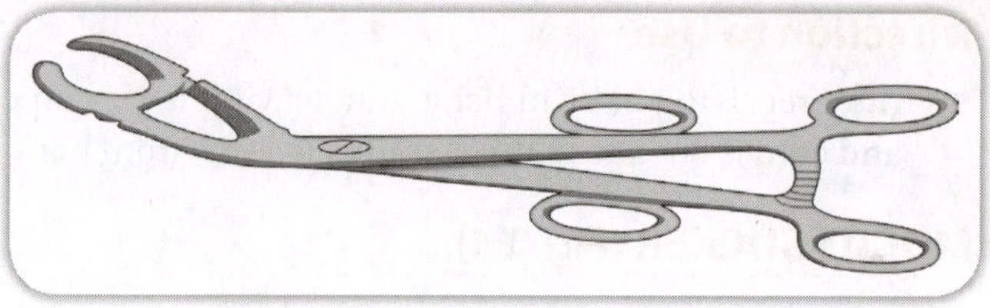

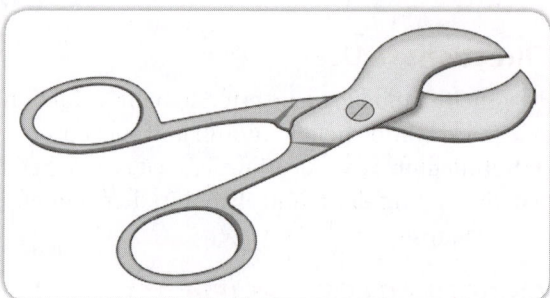

Fig. 26: Bonney's myomectomy clamp

Directions to Use

- Instrument is applied with the angle downward so that the blades go into the pelvis over the pubes while the handles remain horizontal between patient's thigh.
- The instrument is used to achieve temporary compression of the uterine blood vessels so as to reduce intraoperative blood loss. The clamp has to be released for 10 minutes after every 20 minutes of application to prevent uterine anoxic effect.

CORD CUTTING SCISSORS (Fig. 27)

Features

This instrument is made of stainless steel. It is 10.5 cm long. Its blades are so curved that on closing they meet at their tips leaving a gap between.

Uses

- To cut umbilical cord.
- To prevent neonatal infection by using separate scissors for umbilical cord cutting.

Fig. 27: Cord cutting scissors

Directions to Use

- Cord slips when cut with ordinary scissors because it contains Wharton's jelly and it is covered by smooth amniotic membranes.
- Umbilical cord is held in sharp curvature of scissors and a sharp cut is given.

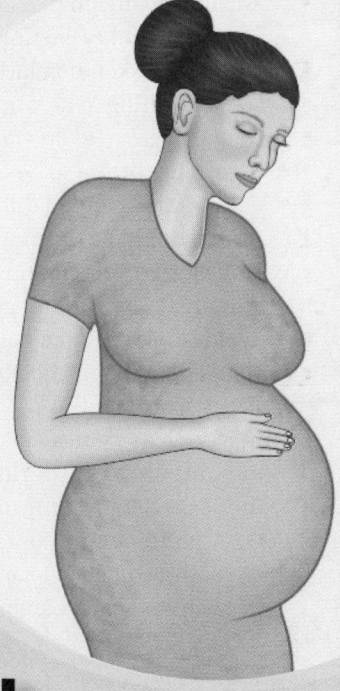

HEALTH ADVICES

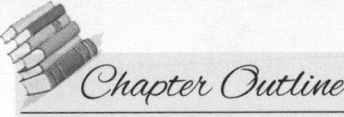

Chapter Outline

- Antenatal Advices
- Antenatal Diet
- Exercises During Pregnancy
- Daily Fetal Kick Monitoring
- Preparation for Labor and Delivery
- Postnatal Advices
- Family Planning Advices
- Postnatal Exercises Advices
- Breastfeeding Techniques Advices
- Kangaroo Mother Care
- Teaching Self Breast Examination

ANTENATAL ADVICES

- A balanced diet to meet the demand of increased calorie requirements.
- Rest and sleep to ensure that the mother is not having discomfort.
- Bath to be taken regularly and avoid slipping in the bathroom.
- Loose clothing to be worn and avoid the high heels shoes.
- Dental hygiene to be maintained and dentist to be consulted earlier.
- Care of the breast to be done by checking any problem in the mothers nipples and treat the same.
- Coitus to be avoided during first and third trimesters of pregnancy.
- Drugs should be taken with caution as almost all the drugs cross the placenta and reach the fetus.
- Traveling by vehicles having jerks should be avoided in the first and the last trimester.
- Immunization with tetanus toxoid is given to give protection to the mother as well as the fetus.
- Avoid smoking and alcohol as it affects the health status of the fetus.
- Regular antenatal check-up positively on the schedule date of visit.
- She is instructed to report to the physician even at an early date if some untoward symptoms arise such as intense headache, disturbed sleep with restlessness, urinary trouble, epigastric pain, vomiting and scanty urination.
- She is advised to come to hospital, if there is
  - Painful uterine contraction.
  - Sudden gush of watery fluid per vaginum.
  - Active vaginal bleeding.

ANTENATAL DIET

PRINCIPLES

- To counsel the women about the importance of regular check-up.
- To maintain or improve the health status of the woman to the optimum till delivery by judicious advice regarding diet, drug and hygiene.
- To improve the psychology and to remove the fear of the unknown by counseling the woman.

DIET

It should be adequate to provide

- Good maternal health.
- Optimum fetal growth.
- The strength and vitality during labor.
- Successful lactation
  - The increased calorie requirement is to extent of 300 over the no pregnancy state during second half of pregnancy.
  - Diet in pregnancy should be of woman's choices.
  - The pregnancy diet ideally should be light, nutritious, easily digestible and rich in protein, mineral and vitamins.
  - Half liter, if not, 1 liter of milk (contains about 1 g of calcium), plenty of green vegetables and fruits.
  - Dietetic advice should be given with due consideration to the socioeconomic condition, food habits and taste of the individual.

- Supplementary iron therapy is needed for all pregnant mothers from 16 weeks onwards.
- 1 table of ferrous sulfate containing 60 mg elemental iron is enough.
- Intake of protein 60 g sources are meat fish, poultry and dairy product.
- Iron rich foods, vitamins, folic acid rich in leafy vegetables and liver. Additionally 1 tab contains 5 mg.

EXERCISES DURING PREGNANCY

ANTENATAL EXERCISES

Benefits

- Muscles of good tone are more elastic and will regain their farther strength more efficiently and more quickly after being stretched than muscles of poor tone.
- Exercising abdominal muscles antenatally will ensure a speedy return to normal postnatally effective pushing in labor gives less backache in pregnancy.
- The ligaments around the pelvis stretch and no longer give such firm support to the joints; the muscles become the second line of defense helping to prevent an exaggerated pelvic tilt and the unnecessary stress on the pelvic ligaments.

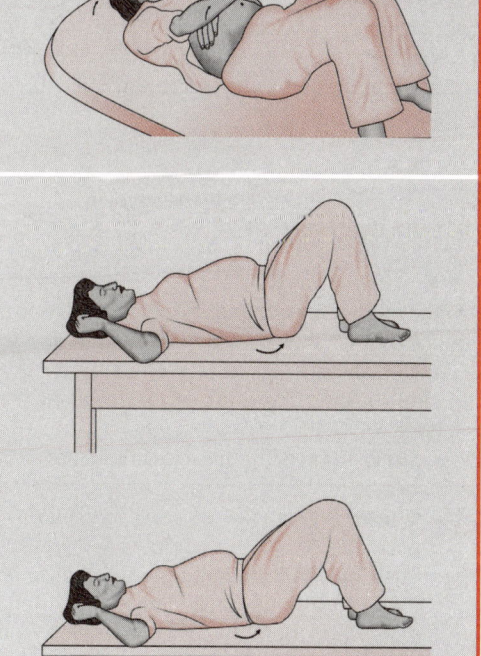

Head Lift with Pelvic Tilt

Steps

- The arms are closed over the diastases and pulled toward midline
- Slowly lift the head off the floor while performing a posterior pelvic tilt, slowly lower the head and relax
- All abdominal contractions should be performed with an exhalation so that intra-abdominal pressure is minimized.

Leg Sliding

Steps

- Hook lying with pelvis in a posterior tilt
- Instruct the woman to hold the pelvic tilt as she first slides one foot along the floor until the leg is straight
- She stops sliding at a point at which she can no longer hold the pelvic tilt. Slowly tilt the leg and bring back to the starting position
- Repeat with other leg. Breathing should be coordinated with the exercise, so that abdominal contractions occur with inhalations.
- This exercise can be performed with both legs at the same time only if abdominal muscles can maintain the pelvic tilt through the entire exercises.

Pelvic Tilt Exercise

Steps

- Quadrupled (on hands and knees) instruct the mother to perform a posterior pelvic tilt while keeping her back straight, have her draw in and tighten the abdomen and hold, then relax and perform an anterior tilt through partial range.

Pelvic Tilting

- Pelvic tilting is useful in strengthening abdominal muscle tone and in reducing low back pain due to postural changes that commonly occurs as the uterus enlarges.

Steps

- Ask women to lie flat on her back with her knees bent and her feet flat on the floor.
- Slowly the woman decreases the lumbar curve by tilting the pelvis to press the small of her back against the floor while simultaneously tighten her abdominal and buttock muscles.
- This exercise should be repeated several times, it can also be done in a standing position using a wall as the flat surface.

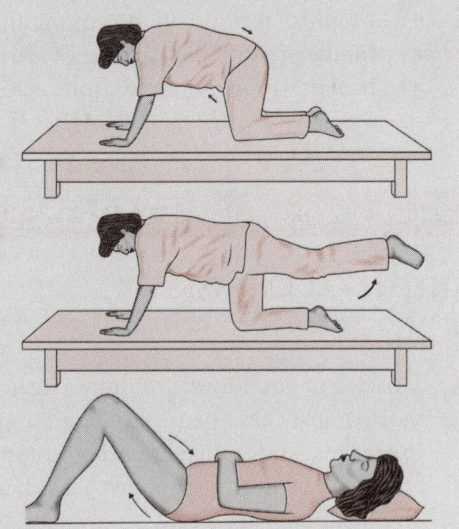

Abdominal Tightening

Steps

- Sit comfortably or kneel on four
- Breathe in and out then pull in the lower part of the abdomen below the umbilicus while continuing to breathe normally
- Hold for up to 10 seconds. Repeat up to 10 times. This tones the deep transverse abdominal muscles which are the main postural support of the spine and will help to prevent back ache in future.

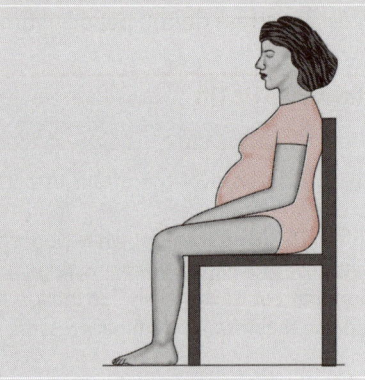

Kegel's Exercise

Steps

- The mother is encouraged doing kegel's exercises
- The mother should locate the muscles and should stop the stream of urine
- After locating the muscles the following exercise can be done.
  - **Slow:** Tighten the muscle, hold it for 3–5 seconds and relax it
  - **Quick:** Tighten the muscle, and relax it as rapidly as possible
  - **Push out, pull in:** Pull up entire pelvic floor as though trying to suck up water into vagina. Then bear down as if trying to push the imaginary water out. Abdominal muscles also involved in this process.

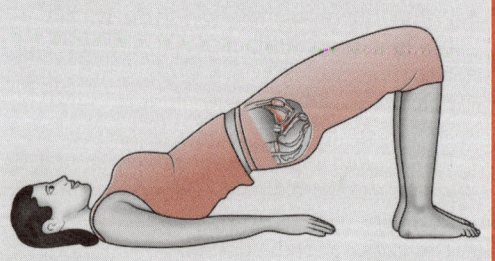

- The exercise can be done 10 times in a row at least three times a day. Good time to practice is during trips to the bathroom, but additional practice at other times is even more beneficial.

Foot and Leg Exercise

The circulation during pregnancy particularly the venous return is sluggish and this can lead to problems such as cramps, varicose veins and edema. To prevent following exercises can be done.

Steps

- Sit or half lie with legs supported
- Bend and stretch the ankles at least 12 times circles both feet at the ankle at least 20 times in each direction.
- Brace both knees, hold for a count of four, then release. Repeat 12 times.

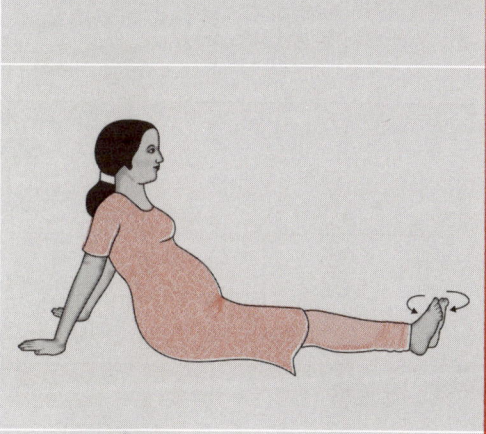

Breathing Awareness

Steps

- Sit comfortably with eyes closed
- Listen into your breathing concentrating especially on the outward breath which naturally follows
- Keep the movement fairly low down in the chest and be aware of your own breathing rate while resting

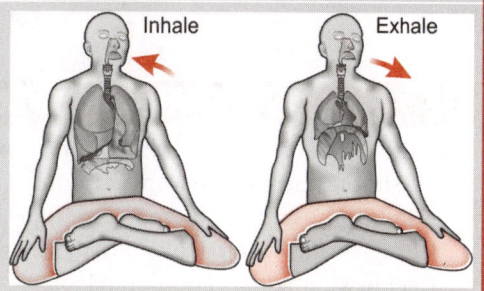

DAILY FETAL KICK MONITORING

Fetal movement count can be done by two methods.

CARDIFF COUNT 10 FORMULA

The patient counts fetal movements starting at 9 am. The counting comes to an end as soon as 10 movements are perceived.

She is instructed to report the physician if:

- Less than 10 movements occur during 12 hours on 2 successive days.
- No movement is perceived even after 12 hours in a single day.

DAILY FETAL MOVEMENT COUNT (DFMC) (Fig. 1)

- Three counts each of 1 hour duration (morning, noon and evening) are recommended.
- The total counts multiplied by four gives daily (12 hour) fetal movement count (DFMC).
- If there is diminution of the number of kicks to less than 10 in 12 hours (or less than 3 in each hour), it indicates fetal compromise.
- Mother perceives 88% of the fetal movements detected by Doppler imaging.
- The count should be performed daily starting at 28 weeks of pregnancy.
- **Loss of fetal movements** is commonly followed by disappearance of fetal heart rate within next 24 hours.

- **Maternal perception of fetal movements may be reduced** with fetal sleep (quiet), fetal anomalies (CNS), anterior placenta, hydramnios, obesity, drug (narcotics), chronic smoking and hypoxia.

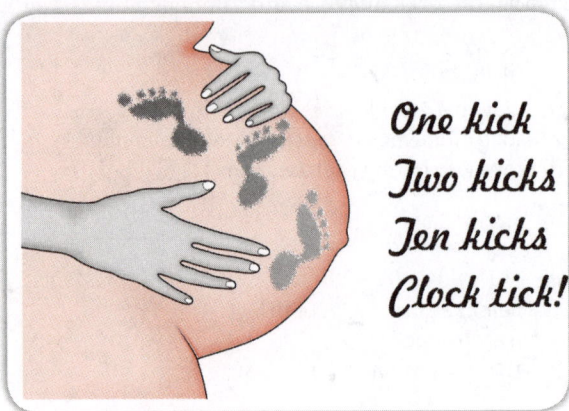

One kick
Two kicks
Ten kicks
Clock tick!

Fig. 1: Fetal kick monitoring

PREPARATION FOR LABOR AND DELIVERY

- Practice the breathing and relaxation exercise regularly.
- Do simple and routine work at home.
- Admit in hospital, if there is any signs of uterine contraction pain increase in regular intervals, leakage from vagina or any bloody discharge.
- Decide whether any additional labor support is required.
- If previously had a cesarean birth, talk with the health care provider about a vaginal birth after a cesarean (VBAC).
- Create the birth plan.
- Make the packing list and pack the labor bag and suitcase.
- Learn the best routes to the hospital.
- Take a childbirth preparation class.
- Consider options for professional birth coaches, such if client and partner decide to seek labor support aside from your health care team.
- Register for a now brother or new sister. Take class to help older children feel better prepared for a hospital trip.

POSTNATAL ADVICES

ADVICES FOR MOTHER AND BABY DURING HOSPITAL STAY

For Mother

- Adequate rest and sleep.
- Should take plenty of oral fluids.
- High protein- and iron-rich diet.
- Light diet should be taken immediately and later well-balanced diet.
- Do not lie on cross. Lie with close legs.

- Observe the vital signs and excessive bleeding report sos.
- Encourage the patient for frequent urination.
- Advice for breast care (clean the breast before and after each breastfeeding).
- Advice for perineal care very often (clean from unclean to clean area).
- Ambulation can be started from 2nd day of postpartum.
- Postnatal exercises.
- Prone position is recommended in between and care of after pain.
- Care of bowel (avoidance of constipation).

For Baby

- Examine the newborn head to toe.
- Keep the baby clean, dry and warm.
- Observe the vomiting, cord bleeding, color, cry, activity, passing of urine and meconium.
- Use the clothes according to the climate.
- Breast feed the baby as early as possible and exclusive breastfeeding.
- Special cord and eye care is given.
- Record the weight of the baby.
- Observe for physiological jaundice and transitional stool.
- Give baby bath after 48 hours or as hospital policy.

ADVICES ON DISCHARGE

For Mother

Do's

- Adopt small family norms.
- Attend postnatal clinic after 6 weeks.
- Follow regular intake of medicines.

Don'ts

- Lifting heavy weights.
- Long journey.
- Sexual intercourse for 6–8 weeks.
- Constipation and strain on sutures especially while sitting.

For baby

Do's

- Immunization as per schedule.
- Attend well baby clinic after 6 – 8 weeks.
- Expose the baby to sunlight for 10–15 minutes every day protecting the eyes.
- Introduced solid food after 6 months.

Don'ts

- Home hazards another infection.
- Top feeds or solid for 6 months.

Postures and posture care

Always keep good posture for
Comfort and good health
To avoid backache, tiredness, sleep problems and leg pain
- Changing weight and hormonal changes affect postures
- Avoid typical pregnancy posture
- Use abdominal and buttock muscles support uterus

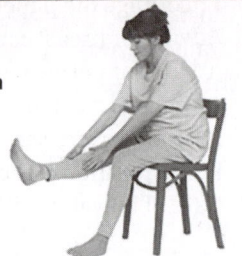

Standing posture
- Tuck in your chin
- Lift shoulders
- Abdomen pulled up
- Back upright and pelvis centered
- Distribute weight evenly on both legs

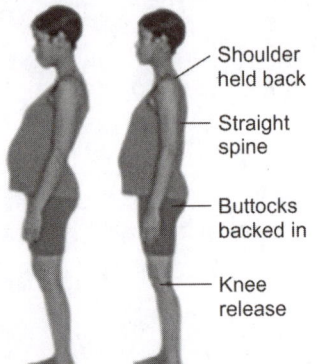

- Shoulder held back
- Straight spine
- Buttocks backed in
- Knee release

Sleeping on side
- Lie on any one side
- Soft pillow under head
- Lower leg straight
- Support abdomen on soft pillow
- Bend upper knee and place on pillow

Correct sitting
- Sit on a straight-backed chair
- Support lower back (use cushion)
- Do not cross legs
- Use footrest

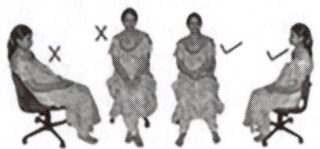

Working/lifting weight
- Do not bend from waist
- Keep back straight
- Bend knees and squat down
- Lift object and stand up
Avoid lifting heavy weight

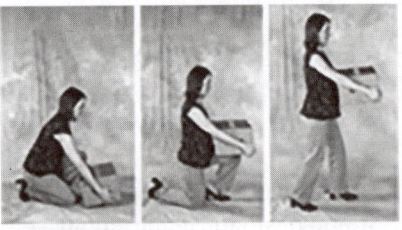

Sleeping on the back
- Soft pillow under head
- Keep pillow under thighs and knees
- Roll legs and feet outwards
In late pregnancy avoid remaining flat on back

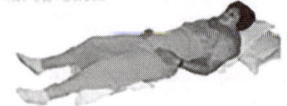

Remember to keep Good posture all the time - day and night

Getting out of bed
- Roll on side
- Bend knees
- Take support of arms and pull body up

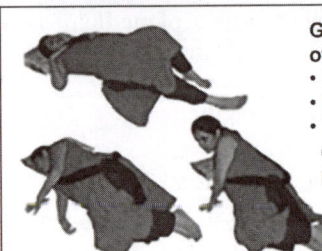

FAMILY PLANNING ADVICES

Breastfeeding

- Is a natural method of family planning.
- Gives 99% security for first 6 months in exclusively breastfeed mothers.
- No guarantee as contraception in non breast feeding mothers.

Cervical Mucus Study (Fig. 2)

- Post period day no count to be kept.
- Daily cervical mucus to be studied for consistency.
- In fertile period mucus is watery and in nonfertile it is thick.
- Coitus is limited to alternate day in nonfertile/safe period in order to avoid confusion in assessing cervical mucus.

Calendar Method (Fig. 3)

- For following this method, one should have regular periods.
- 11–18 days in regular 28–30 days cycles consider as fertile.
- So, coitus in this period to be avoided.
- Lady can mark days in calendar to avoid any confusion.

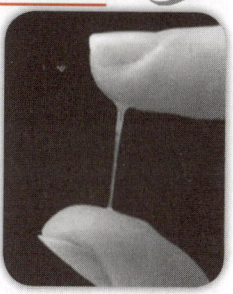

Fig. 2: Cervical mucus being for checked consistency

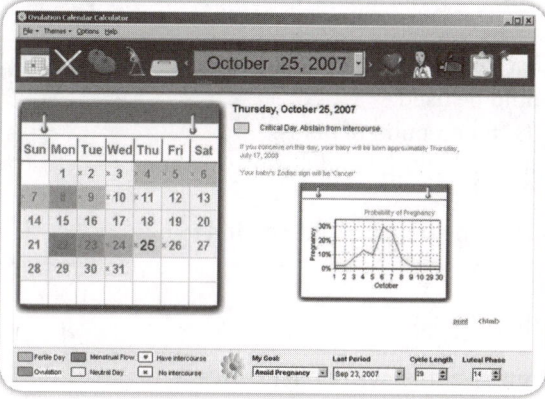

Fig. 3: Calendar method

Basal Body Temperature (Fig. 4)

- Daily axillary temperature to be monitor in morning time.
- It should be plotted in chart.
- 0.5° rise in temperature to be noted (ovulation) and coitus to be avoided.
- If not done properly or with recording errors, pregnancy can occur.

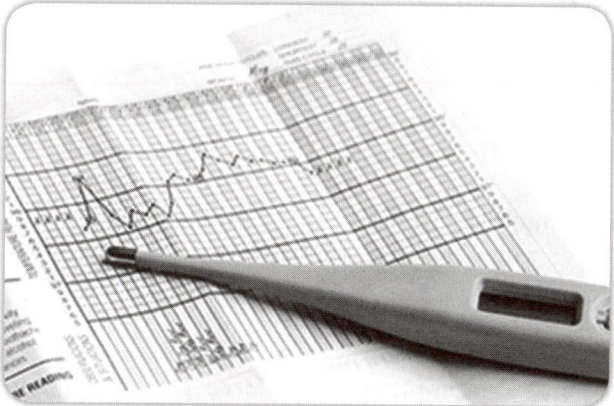

Fig. 4: Temperature monitoring

Abstinence

- It is no coitus at all.
- It provides 100% guarantee of contraception, but difficult to practice.
- Not useful for long term practice.

Coitus Interruptus

- In this penis should be withdrawn from vagina before ejaculation.
- Risk of pregnancy with pre-ejaculatory secretions is present.
- Also, if withdrawal is not done on time risk of pregnancy exists.
- In doubtful cases, emergency contraception is advised.

Condom/Barrier Methods (Fig. 5)

- It is available free of cost at government hospitals and centers.
- It gives protection against sexually transmitted diseases.
- Each time new pack should be used.
- It should be applied just after erection of penis.
- Should be removed, wrapped in paper and dispose of after use.
- If it fails (tears) during use, emergency contraception to be used.

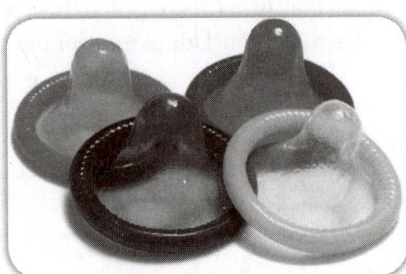

Fig. 5: Condoms

Oral Contraceptive Pills (Fig. 6)

- To follow this method, one should have regular cycles.
- Should start on 2nd day of cycle.
- One tablet each night should be taken.
- Tablets to be taken as per the direction of arrow on wrapper
- Never miss the dose.
- If dose is missed, it should be taken as soon as the person remembers.
- If more than 2 doses are missed, emergency contraception should be used.
- Should not be followed by breastfeeding mothers up to 6 months.

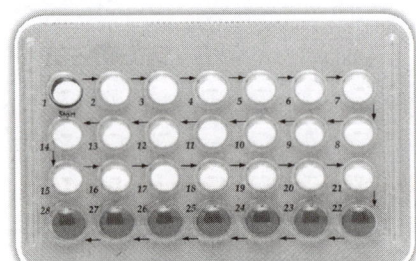

Fig. 6: Oral contraceptive pills

Emergency Contraception (Fig. 7)

- Should not be used on routine basis.
- Can lead to complications like unovulatory cycle, polycystic ovarian syndrome (PCOS) or infertility.
- If use, it is to be taken within 72 hours.
- If taken within 12 hours of coitus, result is favorable.
- Tablet to be taken after food.
- If vomited, to be taken again.
- It can give symptoms like colicky pain in lower abdomen and spotting.
- If regular menses are missed or in presence of above signs for long, ultrasonography to be done.

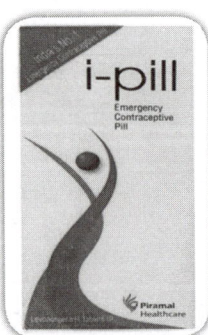

Fig. 7: Emergency contraceptive pills

Intrauterine Devices (IUDs) (Fig. 8)

- Proper perineal hygiene to be maintained.
- Women can have dysmenorrhea and heavy periods.
- At least once a month after menses thread of IUD to be felt.
- If unable to feel to be reported to physician.
- If menses missed by more than a month, urine pregnancy test (UPT) and sonography to be done.
- Report danger signs like very heavy bleeding, prolonged periods and continuous abdominal pain.

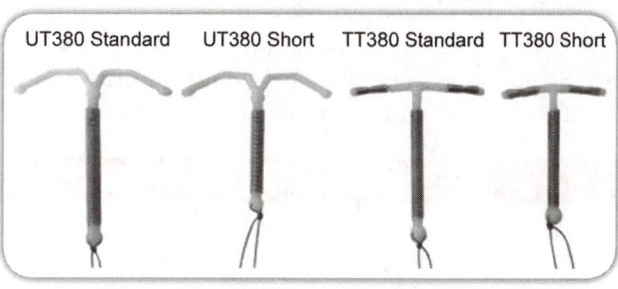

UT380 Standard UT380 Short TT380 Standard TT380 Short

Fig. 8: Different types of Intrauterine Devices

Tubectomy (Fig. 9)

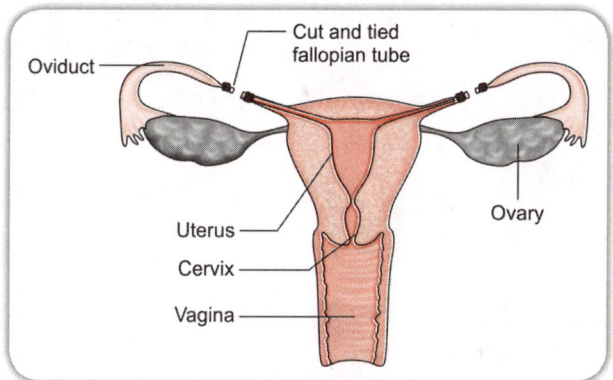

Oviduct

Cut and tied fallopian tube

Uterus

Ovary

Cervix

Vagina

Fig. 9: Tubectomy

- Ensures permanent contraception but in failure case pregnancy can occur.
- If periods are missed for more than a month, UPT and sonography to be done.

Vasectomy (Fig. 10)

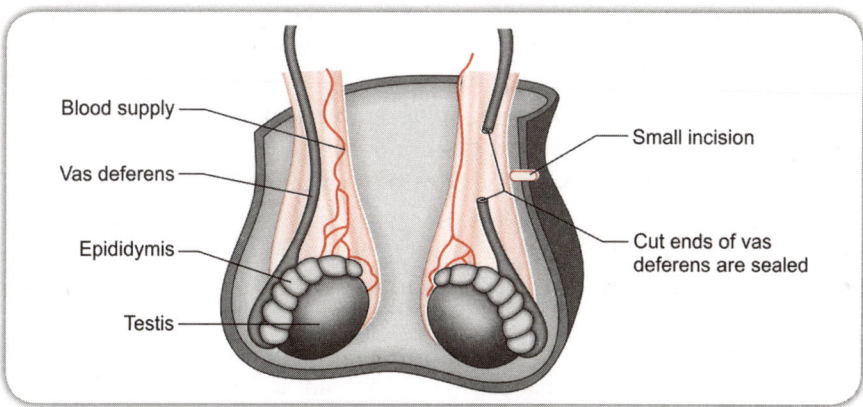

Blood supply

Vas deferens

Epididymis

Testis

Small incision

Cut ends of vas deferens are sealed

Fig. 10: Vasectomy

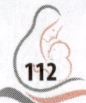

- Most easy and day care procedure.
- Does not requires hospitalization.
- Scrotal support by well-fitting undergarment.
- Barrier precautions to be used for 3 months after surgery.

POSTNATAL EXERCISES ADVICES (Fig. 11)

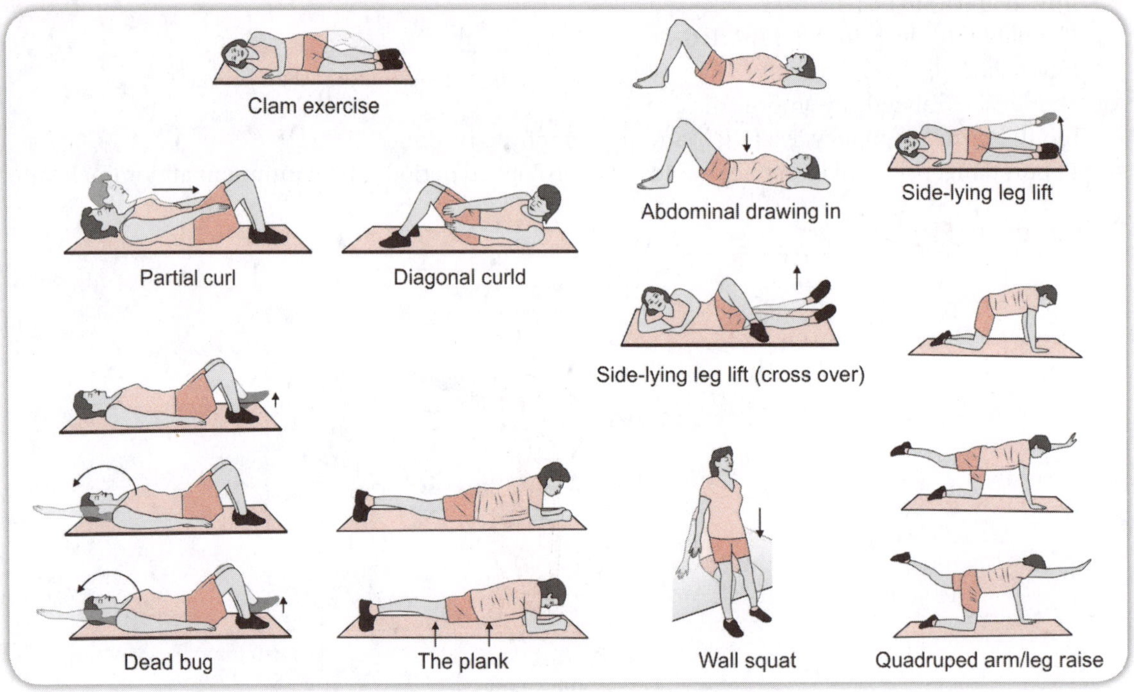

Clam exercise

Partial curl

Diagonal curld

Abdominal drawing in

Side-lying leg lift

Side-lying leg lift (cross over)

Dead bug

The plank

Wall squat

Quadruped arm/leg raise

Fig. 11: Stretching and strengthening exercise after delivery

GENTLE TUMMY EXERCISE

- Pregnancy splits abdominal muscles down the middle. It is important to make sure that muscles should have healed before any vigorous abdominal exercises, such as abdominal crunches.
- In the meantime, tone tummy by performing an exercise that strengthens the deepest muscle layer (transverses abdominus). These exercises can be done in lying down, sitting, and standing position.
  - Keep lower back flat.
  - Breathe out and draw belly back toward spine. Lower back should not flex or move.
  - Hold this position and breathe lightly. Count 1 to 10.
  - Relax and repeat up to 10 times per set. Can do 10 sets per day.

TUMMY EXERCISE – STAGE TWO

Once the gap in abdominal muscles has closed, can progress to more demanding exercises of tummy. General guidelines include:

- Lie on back, with bent knees and both feet on the floor. Put hands on thighs.
- Breathe out, contract your abdominal muscles and lift head and shoulders off the floor. Slide hands toward knees. Only aim to get your shoulder blades off the floor.

- Keep head and shoulders stable. Hold the position and then slowly ease shoulders and head back to the floor.
- Repeat up to 10 times for one set.

EXERCISE FOR THE LOWER ABDOMINAL MUSCLES

Guidelines include:

- Make sure abdominal muscles have healed. Until the gap is closed.
- Lie on back with knees bent and both feet flat on the floor.
- Contract abdominal muscles.
- Slowly slide feet away, aiming to straighten both legs. The idea is to straighten the legs without arching lower back.
- If back starts to arch, stop and slide feet back toward bottom.
- Aim for 10 repetitions per set.

PELVIC FLOOR EXERCISES

- The pelvic floor muscles are tightly slung between coccyx and the pubic bone, and support the bowel, bladder, uterus and vagina. Childbirth can weaken these muscles and cause problems, such as incontinence, later in life. To begin the excercise, must first direct attention to these muscles. These exercises can be performed lying down, sitting or standing.
- **Try to relax abdominal muscles. Do not bear down or hold breath. Gradually squeeze and increase the tension until have contracted the muscles as hard as you can. Release gently and slowly. Then perform the exercises, which include:**
  - Squeeze slowly and hold for between 5 and 10 seconds. Release slowly. Repeat 10 times.
  - Perform quick, short and hard squeezes. Repeat 10 times.
  - Squeeze, then clear throat or cough lightly. Repeat three times.
  - Aim for five or six sets each day.

GENERAL SUGGESTIONS FOR AEROBIC EXERCISE

- Give sufficient time to heal, particularly if had a cesarean birth.
- Consult with doctor before starting any postnatal exercise.
- Aim for slow, gradual weight loss of around half a kilogram per week.
- Wear a supportive bra.
- Avoid any activities that place stress on the unstable pelvic floor and hip joints until strength and stability has improved. Be careful about activities that require sudden changes in direction.
- Initially, exercise for only five to 10 minutes at a time. Increase the length of workouts gradually.
- Ideally, exercise sessions should eventually last between 30 and 50 minutes.
- Drink plenty of water before, during and after exercise.
- Do not push too hard – if feel breathless, slow down.
- If experienced pain, slow down or stop.

Warning Signs to Slow Down

- Increased fatigue.
- Muscle aches and pains.
- Color changes to lochia (post-partum vaginal flow) to pink or red.

- Heavier lochia flow.
- Lochia starts flowing again after it had stopped.

BREASTFEEDING TECHNIQUES ADVICES (Fig. 12)

- Perform breast hygiene routinely.
- Sit in a relax atmosphere.
- Position self and baby with use of pillows. Hold baby at breast level.
- Hold fingers around the breast in 'U' shape to support the breast.
- Touch nipple to baby's cheek and let baby latch on her own.
- Allow baby to latch maximum areola a baby can.
- Give uninterrupted breastfeeding.
- Support baby firmly.
- Practice various positions of breastfeeding.
- Latch alternatively on each breast for 15–20 minutes.
- After feeding release the latch by using little finger to avoid nipple soreness.
- **In between, wake up the baby by tactile stimulation**.
- Burping should be done after each feed.
- Focus on demand feeding.
- Exclusive breastfeeding for first 6 months.
- Mother can take several snacks in between, if feeling fatigued.

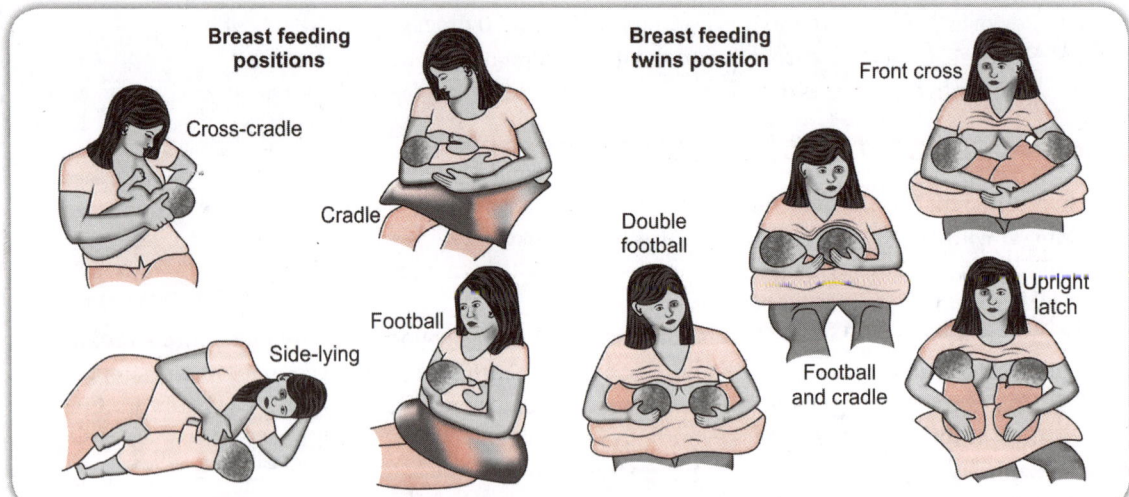

Fig. 12: Techniques of breastfeeding

KANGAROO MOTHER CARE (Fig. 13)

HELP THE MOTHER TO POSITION HER BABY

- Shows the mother the correct position and attachment for breastfeeding.
- **Shows the mother how to hold her baby:** Hold the baby's head and body straight; make the baby face her breast, the baby's nose opposite her nipple; hold the baby's body close to her body; support the baby's whole body, not just the neck and shoulders.
- **Shows the mother how to help her baby to attach:** Touch her baby's lips with her nipple; – wait until her baby's mouth is wide open; move her baby quickly onto her breast, aiming the infant's lower lip well below the nipple.
- **Shows the mother signs of good attachment:** Baby's chin is touching her breast; his mouth is wide open; his lower lip is turned out; a larger area of the areola is visible above rather than below the baby's mouth; suckling is slow and deep, sometimes pausing.

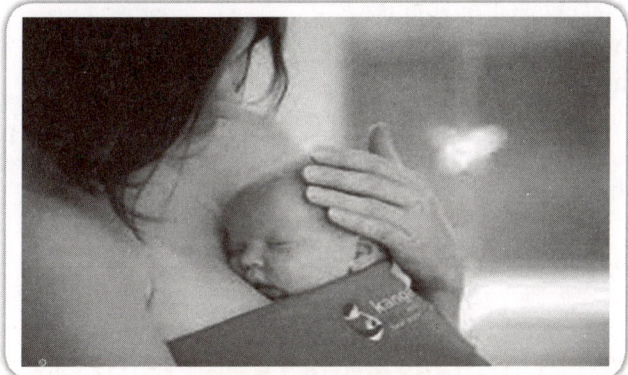

Fig. 13: Kangaroo mother care

THE BABY CAN BE FED WHILE IN KANGAROO POSITION

- Hold the baby in skin-to-skin contact, the mouth close to the nipple.
- Wait until the baby is alert and opens mouth and eyes (very small babies may need light stimulation to be kept awake and alert).
- Express a few drops of breast milk.
- Let the baby smell and lick the nipple, and open the mouth; Express breast milk into the baby's open mouth.
- Wait until baby swallows the milk.
- Repeat the procedure until the baby closes his mouth and will take no more breast milk even after stimulation.
- Ask the mother to repeat this operation every hour if the baby weighs less than 1,200 g and every 2 hours if the baby weighs more than 1,200 g.
- Be flexible at each feed, but check that the intake is adequate by measuring the daily weight gain.

Adequate daily weight gain from the second week of life is 15g/kg/day. Approximate weight gains for different postmenstrual ages are given below:

- 20 g/day up to 32 weeks of postmenstrual age, corresponding approximately to 150–200 g/week.
- 25 g/day from 33 to 36 weeks of postmenstrual age, corresponding approximately to 200–250 g/week.
- 30 g/day from 37 to 40 weeks of postmenstrual age, corresponding approximately to 250–300 g/week.
- Weight babies once a day. Once the baby has started gaining weight, weigh every second day for a week and then once weekly until the baby has reached full term (40 weeks or 2,500 g).
- Weigh the baby in the same way every time, i.e. naked, with the same calibrated scales placing a clean warm towel on the scales to avoid cooling the infant.
- Weigh the baby in a warm environment.
- Growth chart to be maintained.

Mother should return immediately to hospital, if the baby:
- Stops feeding, if not taking well, or vomits.
- Becomes restless and irritable, lethargic or unconscious.
- Has fever (body temperature above 37.5°C);
- Is cold (hypothermia - body temperature below 36.5°C) despite rewarming;
- Has convulsions.
- Has difficulty breathing.
- Has diarrhea.
- Shows any other worrying sign.

TEACHING SELF BREAST EXAMINATION

Purposes
- To assess the own breasts to detect breast carcinoma.
- Breast fibroma.

Equipments Needed
- Mirror.
- Gloves.
- Small pillow or rolled towel.

When it is done?

The best time to do is after the age of 20 years, every month, few days after the menstruation but before 14th day.

PROCEDURE

- Provide privacy and explain the procedure to the patient.
- Wash hands and wear gloves.
- Assist the patient in sitting position facing you and expose chest an breasts.

- Explain and teach breast self-examination as you examine for inspection, ask the patient to stand in front of the mirror and check the both breasts for anything.
- **Step 1:** Begin by looking at your breasts in the mirror with your shoulders straight and your arms on your hips. **(Fig. 14)**
  - Breasts that are their usual size, shape, and color.
  - Breasts that are evenly shaped without visible distortion or swelling.
  - Dimpling, puckering, or bulging of the skin.
  - A nipple that has changed position or an inverted nipple (pushed inward instead of sticking out).
  - Redness, soreness, rash or swelling.

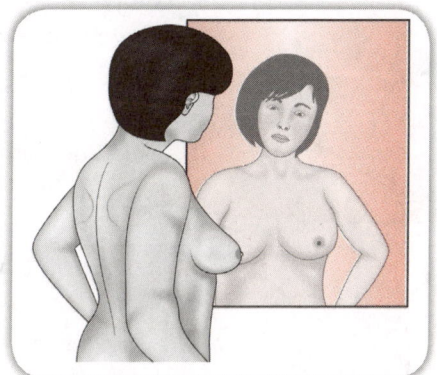

Fig. 14: Examine the breasts in front of mirror

- **Step 2:** Now, raise your arms and look for the same changes. **(Fig. 15)**
- **Step 3:** While you are at the mirror, look for any signs of fluid coming out of one or both nipples (This could be a watery, milky or yellow fluid or blood).

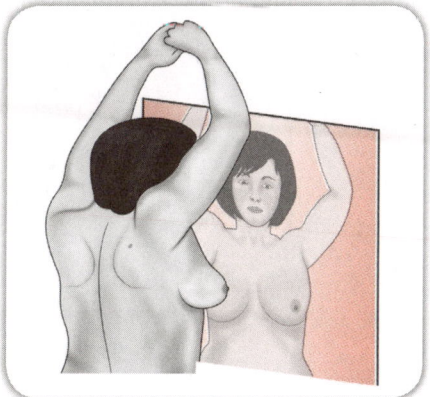

Fig. 15: Examine by raising the hands

- **Step 4:** Next, feel your breasts while lying down, using your right hand to feel your left breast and then your left hand to feel your right breast Use a firm, smooth touch with the first few finger pads of your hand, keeping the fingers flat and together. Use a circular motion or any method. **(Fig. 16)**

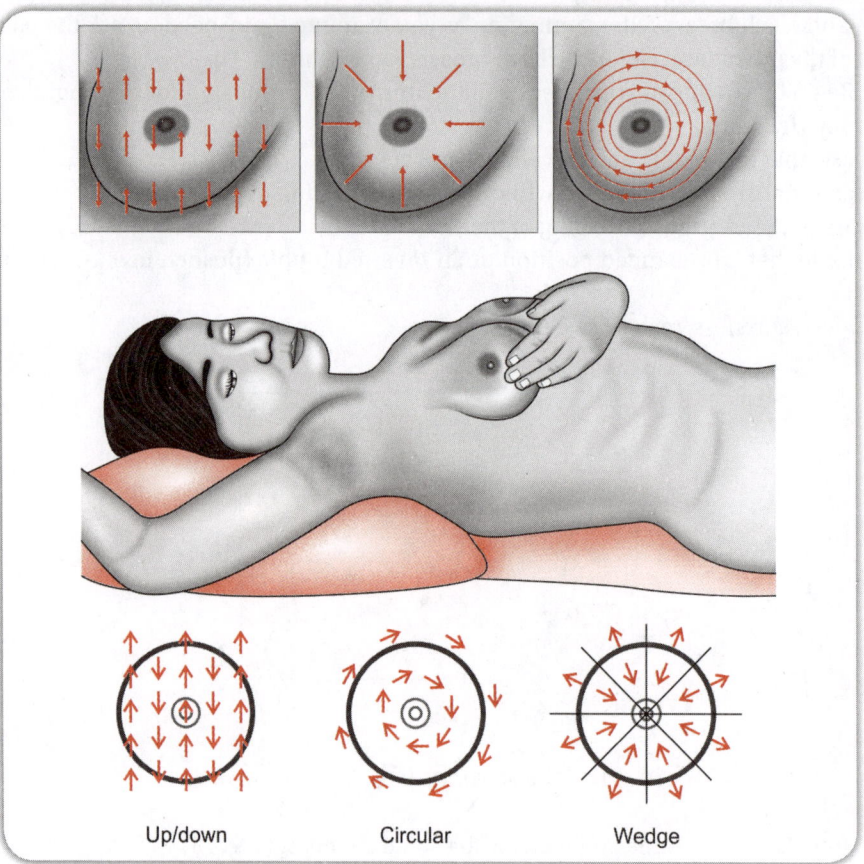

Fig. 16: Examine by movements of hands on breasts

- Repeat on another breast.
- Record and reporting the findings (i.e. tenderness, nipple discharge, hardness in breast and any presence of lump).

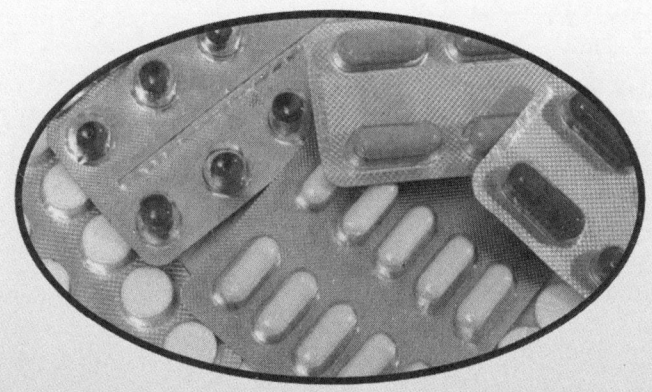

DRUGS USED IN OBSTETRICS

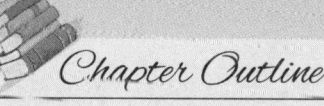

Chapter Outline

OXYTOCIN

Classification

Therapeutic: Hormones
Pharmacologic: Oxytocics

Action

- Stimulates uterine smooth muscle, producing uterine contractions similar to those in spontaneous labor
- It has vasopressor and antidiuretic effects.

Therapeutic effects

- Induction of labor
- Control of postpartum bleeding.

Routes and Doses

- **In induction or stimulation of labor**
  - **Adults:** 0.5–2 milliunits/minutes (IV); increase the dose by 1–2 milliunits/min q 15–60 min until pattern established, then decrease the dose
- **In postpartum hemorrhage:**
  - **Adults:** 10 units infused at 20–40 milliunits/min (IV)
  - **Adults:** 10 units after delivery of placenta (IM)
- **In incomplete or inevitable abortion:**
  - **Adults:** 10 units at a rate of 20–40 milliunits/min (IV).

Availability

Solution for injection: 10 units/mL.

Indications

IV: Induction of labor at term, facilitation of threatened abortion
IV, IM: Postpartum control of bleeding after expulsion of the placenta.

Contraindications

- Hypersensitivity
- Anticipated nonvaginal delivery, cardiac disease and hypovolemic state
- Grandmultipara, contracted pelvis, hysterotomy, malpresentation, fetal distress, obstructed labor

Side Effects

Maternal

- **Central nervous system (CNS):** Coma and Seizures
- **Cardiovascular (CV):** Hypotension, hypochloremia, hyponatremia and water intoxication
- **Miscellaneous:** Increased uterine motility, uterine hyperstimulation, uterine rupture, painful contractions, abruption placentae, decreased uterine blood flow and hypersensitivity.

Fetal

- **CNS:** Intracranial hemorrhage
- **Respiratory:** Asphyxia and hypoxia
- **CV:** Arrhythmias.

Nursing Assessment and Management

- Assess fetal maturity, presentation and pelvic adequacy prior to administration of oxytocin for induction of labor
- Assess character, frequency and duration of uterine contractions; resting uterine tone, maternal pulse, blood pressure and fetal heart rate frequently throughout the administration
- Keep drug $MgSO_4$ ready, if needed for myometrium contraction
- Do not administer oxytocin simultaneously more than one route
- Advice patient to expect contractions similar to menstrual cramps after administration has started
- Explain side effects of the drug and advice patient to report it to health care professional, if they occur.

METHERGINE

Classification

- **Therapeutic:** Oxytocic
- **Pharmacologic:** Ergot alkaloids

Action

Directly stimulates uterine and vascular smooth muscle.

Therapeutic effect

Uterine contraction

Routes and Doses

Adults: 200–400 mcg (0.4–0.6 mg) q6–12 hour for 2–7 days (PO)
Adults: 2,000 mcg (0.2 mg) q 2–4 hour for up to 5 doses (IM, IV)

Indications

Prevention and treatment of postpartum or postabortion hemorrhage caused by uterine atony or subinvolution.

Contraindication

- Contraindicated in hypersensitivity, should not be used to induce labor
- Use cautiously in hypertensive or eclamptic patients, severe hepatic or renal disease, sepsis
- Exercise extreme caution in third stage of labor.
- Suspected pleural pregnancy, organic cardiac disease, Rh negative mother and organic cardiac disease.

Side Effects

- **CNS:** Dizziness, headache
- **Eye, Ear, Nose and Throat (EENT):** Tinnitus
- **Respiratory:** Dyspnea,
- **Cardiovascular (CV):** Hypertension, arrhythmias, chest pain and palpitations
- **Gastrointestinal (GI):** Nausea and vomiting
- **Genitourinary (GU):** Cramps
- **Derma:** Diaphoresis
- **Miscellaneous:** Allergic reaction and gangrene of the toes.

Nursing Assessment and Management

- Minor blood pressure, heart rate and uterine response. Notify health care professional promptly if uterine relaxation becomes prolonged or if character of vaginal bleeding changes
- Assess for signs of ergotism (cold, numb fingers and toes, chest pain, nausea vomiting headache, muscle pain and weakness)
- If no response to methergine, calcium levels may need to be assessed. Effectiveness of medication is decreased with hypocalcemia
- May cause decrease in serum prolactin levels.

EPIDOCIN

Classification

- **Therapeutic:** Smooth muscle relaxant, oxytocic, and antispasmodic
- **Pharmacologic:** Anticholinergics (Antimuscarinic).

Action

Valethamate is an anticholinergic drug used as smooth muscle relaxant. It has both central and peripheral action. It is a competitive inhibitor of ACE. It is used for cervical dilation, gastrointestinal tract spasm, stones. It works by resisting the levels of certain chemicals thus relaxing the smooth muscles of cervix and intestine.

Routes and Doses

- **Adults:** Tablet Valethamate bromide 10 mg and paracetamol 325 mg. 1 tablet 3 times/day (PO)
- **IV/IM:** 8–16 mg/day.

Indications

This medication is an antispasmodic agent; prescribed for dysmenorrhea, GI Spasm, postoperative pain, tenesmus (incomplete defecation) urinary tract and bile stone colic.

Contraindication

Increased eye pressure, benign prostatic hyperplasia, intestinal obstruction, ulcer and hypersensitivity.

Side Effects

- **CNS:** Dizziness
- **EENT:** Blurred vision and dilatation of pupil
- **Mouth:** Difficulty in talking and swallowing, dry mouth.
- **GI:** Vomiting and constipation
- **Cardiac:** Abnormal heart rhythm
- **Urogenital:** Urinary retention
- **Miscellaneous:** Mild increase in body temperature.

Nursing Assessment and Management

- Assess the contractions
- Assess the cervical dilatation
- Check for signs of dysmenorrhea
- Monitor the postoperative pain.

DROTIN

Classification

Generic name: Drotaverine
Trade name: Colicure (80 mg), Tavera-M, Samspas (40 mg), Drovet (80 mg)

Action

Drotaverine inhibits phosphodiesterases hydrolyzing cAMP, thereby increasing cAMP concentration, decreasing Ca uptake of the cells and changing the distribution of calcium among the cells. It may also have minor allosteric calcium channel blocking properties.

Route and Dose

Adult: The recommended dose is 40–8 mg 3 times/day (PO).

Indications

The medicine is an antispasmodic, prescribed for pain and dysfunction caused by smooth muscle spasm.

Contraindications

- **Allergy:** This medicine is not recommended for use if you have a known history of allergy to the active component or any other ingredient present with it
- **Severe liver/kidney disease:** This medicine is not recommended for use if you have a severe impairment of liver or kidney function
- **Heart failure:** This medicine is not recommended for use if you have a disease of the heart characterized by insufficient pumping of blood.

Warnings

Pregnancy, breastfeeding, liver disease, kidney disease and hypotension.

Side Effects

Nausea and vomiting; dry mouth; change in pulse rate; dizzziness; headache; difficulty in breathing; allergic skin reaction; swelling of face, lips, eyelids, tongue, hands and feet fall in blood pressure and fainting.

Nursing Assessment and Management

Assessment

- Monitor blood pressure, pulse and respiratory rate prior to and periodically throughout therapy
- Conduct regular assessment of continued need for treatment.

Management

- Take Drotin 80 mg tablet as instructed by the doctor. Follow the instructions as instructed
- Do not take small or large quantities than recommended
- This medicine can be taken with or without food
- An adequate amount of water should be consumed while taking this medicine
- Caution patient to avoid taking alcohol or other CNS depressants concurrently with this medication
- Emphasize the importance of follow-up examinations to determine effectiveness of the medications.

CABERGOLINE

Classification

- **Therapeutic:** Antihyperprolactinemia
- **Pharmacologic:** Dopamine agonists

Action

Inhibits secretion of prolactin by acting as a dopamine agonist.

Route and Dose

Adults: 0.25 mg twice weekly (PO)

Indications

Treatment of hyperprolactinemia.

Contraindications

Hypersensitivity, lactation, uncontrolled hypertension, history of pulmonary, pericardial, valvular or retroperitoneal fibrotic disorders.

Side Effects

- **CNS:** Dizziness, headache, depression, drowsiness, fatigue, vertigo, nervousness and weakness
- **Respiratory:** Pulmonary fibrosis and pleural effusion
- **EENT:** Abnormal vision
- **CV:** Valvular disorders, postural hypotension and hot flashes
- **GI:** Constipation, nausea, vomiting, abdominal pain and dyspepsia
- **GU:** Dysmenorrhea
- **Endocrine:** Breast pain.

Nursing Assessment and Management

Assessment

- Monitor blood pressure before and frequently during initial therapy
- Supervise ambulation
- Evaluate the cardiac status and consider echocardiography periodically
- Monitor signs of valvular disorders (dyspnea, edema, new cardiac murmur)
- Assess for symptoms of parkinson's disease
- Monitor serum prolactin concentrations monthly until normalized (<20 mcg/L in women and <15 mcg/L in men).

Management

- Instruct patient to take medication as directed, take missed doses as soon as possible within 1/2 days
- Advise patient to change position slowly to minimize orthostatic hypotension
- Caution patient to avoid driving and other activities requiring alertness as the medication causes drowsiness and dizziness
- Caution patient to avoid concurrent use of alcohol during therapy
- Emphasize the importance of follow-up.

Instruct patient that if signs (shortness of breath, blurred vision, sudden headache, severe nausea and vomiting) to inform immediately as these are the signs of pituitary tumors.

HEPARIN

Classification

- **Therapeutic:** Anticoagulants
- **Pharmacologic:** Antithrombotics

Action

Potentiates the inhibitory effect of antithrombin on factor Xa and thrombin. In low doses, prevents the conversion of prothrombin to thrombin by its effects on factor Xa. Higher doses neutralize thrombin, preventing the conversion of fibrinogen to fibrin.

Therapeutic effects: Prevention of thrombus formation. Prevention of extension of existing thrombi.

Routes and Doses

- **Adults:** Intermittent bolus—10,000 units, followed by 5,000–10,000 units. Continuous infusion—5,000 units, followed by 20,000–40,000 units infused (IV).
- **Children> 1 year:** Intermittent bolus—50–100 units/kg, followed by 50–100 units/kg. Continuous infusion—loading dose 75 units/kg, followed by 20 units/kg/hour adjust to maintain aPTT of 60–85sec.
- **Neonates and Infants < 1 year:** Continuous infusion—Loading dose 75 units/kg, followed by 28 units/kg/hr, adjust to maintain aPTT of 60–85 sec.
- **Subcut (Adults):** 5,000 units IV, followed by initial subcut dose of 10,000–20,000 units, then 8,000–10,000, units q 8 hour or 15,000–20,000 units q 12 hour.

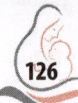

Indications

Prophylaxis and treatment of various thromboembolic disorders including: Venous thrombo-embolism, pulmonary emboli, atrial fibrillation with embolization, acute and chronic consumptive coagulopathies, peripheral arterial thromboembolism. Used in very low doses (10–100 units) to maintain patency of IV catheters.

Contraindications

Hypersensitivity, uncontrolled bleeding, severe actions thrombocytopenia, open wounds, avoid use of products containing benzyl alcohol in premature infants.

Use Cautiously in: Severe liver or kidney disease, retinopathy, untreated hypertension, ulcer disease, spinal cord or brain injury, history of congenital or acquired bleeding disorders, GI bleeding/ulceration/pathology, hemorrhagic stroke, recent CNS or ophthalmologic surgery, active GI bleeding/ulceration, History of thrombocytopenia related to heparin.

Side Effects

- **GI:** Drug-induced hepatitis
- **Dermatology:** Alopecia, rashes and urticaria
- **Hematology:** Bleeding, anemia and thrombocytopenia
- **Local:** Pain at injection site
- **Musculoskeletal (MS):** Osteoporosis
- **Miscellaneous:** Fever and hypersensitivity.

Nursing Assessment and Management

- Assess for signs of bleeding and hemorrhage (bleeding gums, nosebleed, unusual bruising, black tarry stools, hematuria and fall in hematocrit or BP)
- Assess patient for evidence of additional or increased thrombosis. Symptoms will depend on area of involvement
- Monitor patient for hypersensitivity reactions (chills, fever and urticaria)
- **Subcut:** Observe injection sites for hematomas, ecchymosis or inflammation
- Monitor platelet count every 2–3 days throughout therapy.

WARFARIN

Classification

- **Therapeutic:** Anticoagulants
- **Pharmacological:** Coumarins

Action

Interferes with hepatic synthesis of vitamin K-dependent clotting factors.

Therapeutic Effect

Prevention of thromboembolic events.

Routes and Doses

- **Adult:** 2–5 mg/day for 2–4 days (PO, IV)
- **Children>1 month:** 0.2 mg/kg/day for 2–4 days (PO, IV).

Indications

- Prophylaxis and treatment of venous thrombosis, pulmonary embolism, atrial fibrillation with embolization
- Management of myocardial infarction
- Prevention of thrombus formation after the prosthetic valve placement.

Contraindication

- Uncontrolled bleeding, open wounds, active ulcer disease, recent brain, eye or spinal cord injury or surgery
- Uncontrolled hypertension
- Severe liver or kidney disease
- During pregnancy it crosses placenta and may cause fetal hemorrhage. It may also cause congenital malformation.

Note: Use cautiously in malignancy, patient with history of ulcer or liver disease, history of poor compliance, pregnant women.

Side Effects

- **Derma:** Dermal necrosis
- **GI:** Cramps and nausea
- **Hematology:** Bleeding
- **Miscellaneous:** Fever.

Nursing Assessment and Management

Assessment

- Assess for signs of bleeding and hemorrhage (bleeding gums; nosebleed; unusual bruising; tarry, black stools; hematuria; fall in hematocrit or blood pressure; guaiac-positive stools, urine, or nasogastric aspirate)
- Assess for evidence of additional or increased thrombosis. Symptoms depend on area of involvement
- **Geriatrics:** Patients over 60 years exhibit greater than expected prothrombin time/international normalized ratio (PT/INR) response. Monitor for side effects at lower therapeutic ranges.
- **Pediatric:** Achieving and maintaining therapeutic PT/INR ranges may be more difficult in the pediatric patient. Assess PT/INR levels more frequently.
- **Lab test considerations:** Monitor PT, INR and other clotting factors frequently during therapy. Therapeutic PT ranges from 1.3 to 1.5 times greater than control; however, the INR, a standardized system that provides a common basis for communicating and interpreting PT results, is usually referenced. Heparin may affect the PT/INR; draw blood for PT/INR in patients receiving both heparin and warfarin at least 5 hours after the IV bolus dose, 4 hours after cessation of IV infusion, or 24 hours after subcut heparin injection

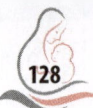

- Monitor hepatic function and CBC before and periodically throughout therapy
- Monitor stool and urine for occult blood before and periodically during therapy
- **Toxicity and overdose:** Withholding 1 or more doses of warfarin is usually sufficient if INR is excessively elevated or if minor bleeding occurs. If overdose occurs or anticoagulation needs to be immediately reversed, the antidote is vitamin K. Administration of whole blood or plasma may also be required in severe bleeding because of the delayed onset of vitamin K.

Implementation

- **High alert:** Medication errors involving anticoagulants have resulted in serious harm or death from internal or intracranial bleeding. Before administering, evaluate recent INR or PT results and have second practitioner should independently check original order.
- Administer medication at same time each day.
- **Postoperative:** Medication requires 3–5 days to reach effective levels; usually begun while patient is still on heparin.
- IV Administration
  - **Direct IV:** Reconstitute each 5–mg vial with 2.7 mL of sterile water for injection. Reconstituted solution is stable for 4 hours at room temperature
  - **Diluent:** No further dilution is needed before administration
  - **Concentration:** 2 mg/mL
  - **Rate:** Administer over 1–2 min.

Family Teaching

- Review foods high in vitamin K. Advise patient to avoid cranberry juice or products during therapy
- Caution patient to avoid IM injections and activities leading to injury. Instruct patient to use a soft toothbrush, not to floss and to shave with an electric razor during warfarin therapy.
- Advise patient to report any symptoms of unusual bleeding or bruising and pain, color or temperature change to any area of your body to health care professional immediately.
- Instruct patient not to drink alcohol or take other Rx, OTC, or herbal products, especially those containing aspirin or NSAIDs, or to start or stop any new medications during warfarin therapy without advice of health care professional
- Advise patient to notify health care professional if pregnancy is planned or suspected or if breastfeeding
- Instruct patient to carry identification describing medication regimen at all times and to inform all health care personnel caring for patient on anticoagulant therapy before lab tests, treatment, or surgery
- Emphasize the importance of frequent lab tests to monitor coagulation factors.

VITAMIN K

Classification

- **Therapeutic:** Antidotes and vitamins
- **Pharmacologic:** Fat-soluble vitamins

Action

Required for hepatic synthesis of blood coagulation factor-II, VII, IX and X

Therapeutic Effect

Prevention of bleeding due to hypoprothrombinemia.

Routes and Doses

- **At birth :** 1 mg IM
- **Children > 1 month:** 1–2 mg (Subcutaneous IV, IM)
- **Children > 1 month:** 2.5–5 mh/day (PO)

Indications

- Prevention and treatment of hypothrombinemia, which may be associated with excessive doses of oral anticoagulants, salicylic, certain anti-infective agents, nutritional deficient and prolonged total parenteral nutrition
- Prevention of hemorrhagic disease of newborn.

Contraindication

Contraindicated in:
- **Hypersensitivity:** Hypersensitivity or intolerance to benzyl alcohol.

Note: Use cautiously in impaired liver function.

Side Effects

- **Derma:** Flushing, rash and urticarial
- **GI:** Gastric upset, unusual taste
- **Hematology:** Hemolytic anemia
- **Local:** Erythema, pain at injection site and swelling
- **Miscellaneous:** Allergic reactions, hyperbilirubinemia, kernicterus.

Nursing Assessment and Management

Assessment

- Monitor for frank and occult bleeding
- Monitor pulse and blood pressure frequently
- **Pediatrics:** Monitor for side effects and adverse reactions. Children may especially be sensitive to the effect and side effect of vitamin k. Neonates, especially premature neonates, may be more sensitive than older children
- **Lab test consideration:** Monitor prothrombin time prior to and throughout therapy.

Implementation

- Administration of whole blood or plasma also be required in severe bleeding because of the delayed onset of this medications
- Vitamin K is antidote for warfarin overdose but does not counteract the anticoagulant activity of heparin.
- **IV administration:**
  - **Direct IV: Diluent:** Dilute with 0.9 % NaCl, D5W
  - **Rate:** 1 mg/min.

Family Teaching

- Instruct the patient to take medicine as directed by physician
- Take next dose as soon as remembered unless almost time for next dose
- Patient should not drastically alter diet while taking vitamin K
- Use soft tooth brush, do not floss, and shave with an electric razor
- Advice patient to report any unusual symptoms of bleeding or brushing
- Advice patient to carry identifications at all times describing disease process
- Emphasize the importance of frequent lab test to monitor the coagulation factor.

RhoGAM

Classification

- **Therapeutic:** Vaccines/immunizing agents
- **Pharmacological:** Immune globulins
  Pregnancy category C

Action

- Prevent production of anti-Rho (D) antibodies in Rho (D)-negative patient who were exposed to Rho (D) positive blood
- Increased platelet counts in patients with idiopathic thrombocytopenic purpura (ITP).

Therapeutic effect

Prevention of antibody response and hemolytic disease of the newborn in future pregnancies of women who have conceived a Rho (D) positive fetus.

Prevention of Rho (D) sensitization following transfusion accident decreases bleeding in patient with ITP.

Route and Dose

Intramuscular use only

Following delivery	**Adult** 300 mcg within 72 hours
Before delivery	**Adult** 300 mcg within 26–28 weeks
Termination of pregnancy	**Adult** 300 mcg within 72 hours
Large fetal – maternal hemorrhage	**Adult** 200 mcg/mL
Transfusion accident	**Adult** 300 mcg

Indications

Administration to Rho (D) –negative patients who have been exposed to Rho (D)-positive by pregnancy or delivery of Rho (D)-positive infant, abortion Rho (D)-positive fetus, fetal –maternal hemorrhage due to amniocentesis, other obstetrical manipulative procedures, or intra-abdominal trauma while carrying Rho (D) –positive fetus, transfusion of Rho (D)-positive blood or blood products to Rho (D)-negative products.

Contraindication

- **Contraindicated in:** Prior hypersensitivity reactions to human immune globin; Rho (D) or du-positive patients.
- **Use cautiously in:** ITP patients with pre-existing anemia.
  May also cause disseminated intravascular coagulation in ITP patient.

Side Effects

- **Skin:** Rash
- **Central nervous system:** Dizziness and headache
- **Cardiovascular system:** Hypertension and hypotension
- **Gastrointestinal system:** Vomiting, diarrhea, nausea
- **Local:** Pain at injection site
- **Musculoskeletal system:** Arthralgia, myalgia
- **Hematology:** ITP, anemia, intravascular hemolysis
- **Miscellaneous:** Fever.

Nursing Assessment and Management

Assessment

- Assess the vital signs during and periodically throughout therapy in patients receiving IV Rho (D) immunoglobulin
- **ITP:** Monitor patient for sign and symptoms of intravascular hemolysis (back pain, shacking, chills, fever, hemoglobinuria), anemia, and renal insufficiency. If transfusions are required use Rho (D)-negative packed red blood cells to prevent exacerbation of intraventricular hemorrhage (IVH)
- **Lab test consideration:** Type and cross match of mother and newborns cord blood must be perform to determine need for medication
- An infant born to a woman treated with Rho (D) immunoglobulin antepartum may have a weekly positive direct combs test result on cord or infant blood
- **ITP:** Monitor platelet count, RBC counts, hemoglobin and reticulocyte levels to determine effectiveness of therapy.

Implementation

- Do not give to infant to Rho (D) positive individual or to Rho (D) negative individual previously sensitized to the Rho (D) antigen
- Do not confused IM and IV formulation. Rh- immunoglobulin for IV administration is labelled "Rh immune globulin intravenous"
- When using prefilled syringes allow solution to reach room temperature before administration

- **IM:** Reconstitute Rho (D) immunoglobulin IV for IM use immediately before use with 1.25 mL of 0.9% of NaCl
- Administer into the deltoid muscle. Dose should be given within 3 hours but may be given up to 72 hours after delivery, miscarriage, abortion and transfusion.
- **IV administration:**
  - **Direct IV diluent:** Dilute with 2.5 mL of 0.9 % of NaCl.
  - **Rate:** 3–5 minutes

Family Teaching

- **Pregnancy:** Explain to patient that the purpose of this medication is to protect future Rho (D)-positive infants
- Explain the purpose of medication to patient.

CEFUROXIME

Classification

- Therapeutic: Anti-infective
- Pharmacologic: Second-generation cephalosporins.

Indications

Treatment of respiratory tract infections, skin and skin structure infections, bone and joint infections (IV), urinary tract infections, gynecological infections, septicemia (IV), otitis media (PO), meningitis (IV), lyme disease (PO). Perioperative prophylaxis (IV).

Action

Binds to bacterial cell wall membrane, causing cell death.

Therapeutic effects: Bactericidal action against susceptible bacteria. Spectrum: Similar to that of first-generation cephalosporins but has increased activity against several other Gram-negative pathogens including: *Haemophilus influenzae* (including β-lactamase-producing strains), *Haemophilus parainfluenzae, Escherichia coli, Klebsiella pneumoniae, Neisseria*, Proteus, *Moraxella catarrhalis, Borrelia burgdorferi*. Not active against methicillin-resistant staphylococci or enterococci.

Contraindications

- **Contraindicated in** hypersensitivity to cephalosporins; Serious hypersensitivity to penicillins.
- **Use cautiously in:** Renal impairment (dose reduction/increased dosing interval recommended if CCr ≤20 mL/min); History of GI disease, especially colitis; Geriatric patients (dose adjustment may be required due to age-related ↓ in renal function); Pregnancy and lactation (has been used safely).

Side Effects

- **Central nervous system:** Seizures (high doses)
- **Gastrointestinal:** Pseudomembranous colitis, diarrhea, nausea, vomiting, cramps
- **Dermatology:** Rashes, urticaria and diaper dermatitis
- **Hematology:** Bleeding, eosinophilia, hemolytic anemia, leukopenia
- **Local:** Pain at IM site, phlebitis at IV site
- **Miscellaneous:** Allergic reactions including anaphylaxis, superinfection.

Interactions

Drug: Probenecid decreases excretion and increases blood levels. Aminoglycosides and loop diuretics may increase the risk of nephrotoxicity.

Routes and Dosages

- **Postoperative (Adults and Children >12 years):** Pharyngitis/tonsillitis, maxillary sinusitis, uncomplicated urinary tract infections—250 mg every 12 hour
- Bronchitis, uncomplicated skin/skin structure infections—250–500 mg every 12 hour. Gonorrhea—1 g single dose. Lyme disease—500 mg every 12 hour for 20 days
- **Postoperative (Children 3 months–12 year):** Otitis media, acute bacterial maxillary sinusitis, impetigo—15 mg/kg every 12 hours as oral suspension (not to exceed 1 g/day) or 250 mg every 12 hours as tablets. Pharyngitis/tonsillitis—10 mg/kg every 12 hour as oral suspension, not to exceed 500 mg/day
- **Adults (IM, IV):** Uncomplicated urinary tract infections, skin/skin structure infections, disseminated gonococcal infections, uncomplicated pneumonia-750 mg every 8 hour. Bone/joint infections, severe or complicated infections—1.5 g every 8 hour. Life-threatening infections-1.5 g every 6 hour. Meningitis-3 g every 8 hour. Perioperative prophylaxis-1.5 g IV 30–60 min before initial incision; 750 mg IM/IV every 8 hour can be given when procedure prolonged. Prophylaxis during open-heart surgery-1.5 g IV at induction of anesthesia and then every 12 hour for 3 additional doses. Gonorrhea—1.5 g IM (750 mg in two sites) with 1g probenecid PO
- **Children and Infants >3 months (IM, IV):** Most infections—50–100 mg/kg/day divided every 6–8 hr (maximum dose 6 g/day). Bone and joint infections—150 mg/kg/day divided every 8 hr (maximum dose 6 g/day)
- Renal Impairment
- **Adults (IM, IV):** CCr 10–20 mL/min—750 mg every 12 hour; CCr<10 mL/min—750 mg every 24 hour.

Nursing Assessment and Management

- Assess for infection (vital signs; appearance of wound, sputum, urine, and stool, WBC) at beginning of and throughout therapy
- Before initiating therapy, obtain a history to determine previous use of and reactions to penicillins or cephalosporins. Persons with a negative history of penicillin sensitivity may still have an allergic response
- Obtain specimens for culture and sensitivity before initiating therapy. First dose may be given before receiving results.
- Observe patient for signs and symptoms of anaphylaxis (rash, pruritus, laryngeal edema, wheezing). Discontinue the drug and notify health care professional immediately if these symptoms occur. Keep epinephrine, an antihistamine, and resuscitation equipment close by in the event of an anaphylactic reaction.
- Monitor bowel function. Diarrhea, abdominal cramping, fever, and bloody stools should be reported to health care professional promptly as a sign of pseudomembranous colitis. May begin up to several weeks following cessation of therapy.

Lab Test Considerations

- May cause positive results for Coombs' test
- May cause ↑ serum AST, ALT, alkaline phosphatase, bilirubin, LDH, BUN and creatinine
- May rarely cause leukopenia, neutropenia and eosinophilia.

Potential Nursing Diagnoses

- Risk for infection (Indications, side effects)
- Diarrhea (Adverse reactions)
- Deficient knowledge, related to medication regimen (Patient/Family Teaching).

METRONIDAZOLE

Classifications

Antimicrobial, Antiprotozoa, Amebicidal

Action

Disrupts DNA and protein synthesis in susceptible organisms

Therapeutic Effects

Bactericidal, trichomonacidal or amebicidal action. Spectrum: Most notable for activity against anaerobic bacteria, including: Bacteroides, *Clostridium*. In addition, it is active against: *Trichomonas vaginalis, Entamoeba histolytica, Giardia lamblia, H. pylori, Clostridium difficile*.

Routes and Dosages

- **Adults (PO): Anaerobic infections—7.5 mg/kg q6hr (not to exceed 4 g/day). Trichomoniasis:** 250 mg q8hr for 7 days or single 2-g dose or 1 g twice daily for 1 day. Amebiasis—500– 750 mg q8hr for 5– 10 days. *H. pylori*—250 mg 4 times daily or 500 mg twice daily for 1– 2 weeks (with other agents). Bacterial vaginosis— 750 mg once daily as ER tablets for 7 days. Antibiotic associated pseudomembranous colitis—250– 500 mg 3– 4 times/day for 10–14 days.
- **Infants and children (PO):** Anaerobic infections—30 mg/kg/day divided q6hr, maximum dose: 4 g/day Trichomoniasis: 15– 30 mg/kg/day divided q8hr for 7– 10 days. Amebiasis—35– 50 mg/kg/day divided q8hr for 5– 10 days (not to exceed 750 mg/dose). Antibiotic associated pseudomembranous colitis—30 mg/kg/day divided q6hr for 7– 10 days. *H. pylori*—15– 20 mg/kg/day divided twice daily for 4 weeks.
- **Neonates 0– 4 weeks, 1200 g (IV, PO):** 7.5 mg/kg q48hr. Postnatal age 7 days, 1, 200– 2, 000 g—7.5 mg/kg/day q2hr. Postnatal age 7 days
  - 2,000 g— 15 mg/kg/day divided q12hr. Postnatal age
  - 7 days, 1,200– 2,000 g—15 mg/kg/day divided q12hr. Postnatal age
  - 7 days, 2,000 g—30 mg/kg/day divided q12hr.
- **Adults (IV):** Anaerobic infections: Initial dose 15 mg/kg, then 7.5 mg/kg q6-8hr or 500 mg q6-8 hr (not to exceed 4 g/day). Perioperative prophylaxis—Initial dose 15 mg/kg 1 hour before surgery, then 7.5 mg/kg 6 and 12 hours later. Amebiasis: 500– 750 mg q8hr for 5– 10 days
- **Children (IV):** Anaerobic infections—30 mg/kg/day divided q6hr, maximum dose: 4 g/day.
- **Topical (Adults):** Acne rosacea: Apply thin film to affected area bid.
- **Vaginal (Adults):** Bacterial vaginosis: One applicatorful (5 g) 2 times daily for 5 days.

Indications

- **PO, IV:** Treatment of the following anaerobic infections: Intra-abdominal infections (may be used with a cephalosporin), Gynecologic infections, skin and skin structure infections, lower respiratory tract infections, bone and joint infections, CNS infections, septicemia, endocarditis. **IV** Perioperative prophylactic agent in colorectal surgery. **PO:** Amebicide in the management of amebic dysentery, amebic liver abscess, and trichomoniasis: Treatment of peptic ulcer disease caused by Helicobacter pylori. **Topical** treatment of acne rosacea. **Vaginal:** Management of bacterial vaginosis.

  Unlabeled use: Treatment of giardiasis. Treatment of anti-infective associated pseudomembranous colitis.

Contraindications

- **Contraindicated in** hypersensitivity, hypersensitivity to parabens (topical only)
- **Obstetrics (OB)** first, trimester of pregnancy
- **Use Cautiously in** history of blood dyscrasias, history of seizures or neurologic problems, severe hepatic impairment (dose suggested)
- **OB:** Although safety not established, has been used to treat trichomoniasis in 2nd- and 3rd-trimester pregnancy— but not as single-dose regimen
- **Lactation:** If needed, use single dose and interrupt nursing for 24 hr thereafter; Patients receiving corticosteroids or predisposed to edema (injection contains 28 mEq sodium/g metronidazole).

Side Effects

- **CNS:** Seizures, dizziness, headache, aseptic meningitis (IV), encephalopathy (IV)
- **EENT:** Optic neuropathy, tearing (topical only)
- **GI:** Abdominal pain, anorexia, nausea, diarrhea, dry mouth, furry tongue, glossitis, unpleasant taste, vomiting
- **Dermatology:** Stevens-Johnson Syndrome, rash, urticarial topical only, burning, mild dryness, skin irritation and transient redness
- **Hemat:** Leukopenia
- **Local:** Phlebitis at IV site
- **Neurology:** Peripheral neuropathy
- **Miscellaneous:** Superinfection.

Nursing Assessment and Management

Assessment

- Assess for infection (vital signs; appearance of wound, sputum, urine, and stool; WBC) at beginning of and throughout therapy
- Obtain specimens for culture and sensitivity before initiating therapy. First dose may be given before receiving results
- Monitor neurologic status during and after IV infusions. Inform health care professional if numbness, paresthesia, weakness, ataxia or seizures occur
- Monitor intake and output and daily weight, especially for patients on sodium restriction. Each 500 mg of premixed injection for dilution contains 14 mEq of sodium

- Assess for rash periodically during therapy. May cause Stevens-Johnson syndrome. Discontinue therapy if severe or if accompanied with fever, general malaise, fatigue, muscle or joint aches, blisters, oral lesions, conjunctivitis, hepatitis and/or eosinophilia
- **Giardiasis:** Monitor three stool samples taken several days apart, beginning 3–4 weeks after treatment
- **Lab test considerations:** May alter results of serum AST, ALT, and LDH tests.

Patient/Family Teaching

- Instruct patient to take medication as directed with evenly spaced times between doses, even if feeling better. Do not skip doses or double upon missed doses. Take missed doses as soon as remembered, if not almost time for next dose
- Advise patients treated for trichomoniasis that sexual partners may be asymptomatic sources of reinfection and should be treated concurrently. Patient should also refrain from intercourse or use a condom to prevent reinfection
- Caution patient to avoid intake of alcoholic beverages or preparations containing alcohol during and for at least 3 days after treatment with metronidazole, including vaginal gel. May cause a disulfiram-like reaction (flushing, nausea, vomiting, headache and abdominal cramps)
- May cause dizziness or light-headedness. Caution patient to avoid driving or other activities requiring alertness until response to medication is known
- Instruct patient to notify health care professional promptly if rash occurs
- Inform patient that medication may cause an unpleasant metallic taste
- Advise patient to notify health care professional of all Rx or OTC medications, vitamins, or herbal products being taken and to consult with health care professional before taking other medications
- Advise patient that frequent mouth rinses, good oral hygiene, and sugarless gum or candy may minimize dry mouth. Notify health care professional if dry mouth persists for more than 2 weeks
- Inform patient that medication may cause urine to turn dark
- Advise patient to consult health care professional if no improvement in a few days or if signs and symptoms of superinfection (black, furry overgrowth on tongue; vaginal itching or discharge; loose or foul-smelling stools) develop
- Advise patient to inform health care professional if pregnancy is suspected before taking this medication or if breast feeding
- **Vag:** Instruct patient in correct technique for intravaginal instillation. Advise patient to avoid intercourse during treatment with vaginal gel
- **Topical:** Instruct patient on correct technique for application of topical gel. Cosmetics may be used after application of gel.

FLUCONAZOLE

Classification

Therapeutic: Antifungals (systemic)

Action

Inhibits synthesis of fungal steroids, a necessary component of the cell membrane
- **Therapeutic Effects:** Fungistatic action against susceptible organisms. May be fungicidal in higher concentration
- **Spectrum:** Cryptococcus neoformans. Candida spp.

Routes and Doses

Oropharyngeal Candidiasis

Adults: 200 mg initially then 100 mg daily for at least 2 weeks (PO, IV)
Children: 6 mg/kg. Initially, then 3 mg/kg/day at least 2 weeks (PO, IV)
Neonates: 5–6 mg/kg/dose q 48–72 hour. (PO, IV)

Esophageal candidiasis

Adults: 200 mg initially then 100 mg once daily for 3 weeks (PO, IV)
Children: 6 mg/kg initially then 3–12 mg/kg/day for 3 weeks (PO, IV)
Neonates: 5–6 mg/kg/dose q 48–72 hour. (PO, IV)

Vaginal candidiasis

Adults: 150 mg single dose; prevention of recurrence_150 mg daily for 3 days (PO, IV)

Systemic candidiasis

Adult: 400 mg/daily initially, then 200–800 mg/day for 28 days (PO, IV)
Children: 6–12 mg/kg/day for 28 days (PO, IV)
Neonates: 5–6 mg/kg/dose q 48–72 hours. (PO, IV)

Cryptococcal Meningitis

- **Adult:** 400 mg once daily until favorable clinical response then 200–800 mg once daily (PO, IV) for 10–12 wks after clearing of CSF
- **Children:** 12 mg/kg/dose q 48–72 hours. (PO, IV)

Indications

- **Fungal infection caused by susceptible organisms, including:** Oropharyngeal or esophageal candidiasis, serious systemic candidal infection, urinary tract infection, peritonitis, cryptococcal meningitis. Prevention of candidiasis in patient who have undergone bone marrow transplantation.
- **Unlabeled use:** Prevention of recurrent vaginal yeast infection.

Contraindications

Hypersensitivity to fluconazole or others azole antifungal; concurrent use with pimozide.

Use cautiously in renal impairement (dose reduction required if CCR50 mL/min); underlying liver disease; OB: Safety not established; lactation: Usually compatible with breast feeding (AAP); Geri: increased risk of adverse reaction (rashes, vomiting, diarrhea and seizures); considered age related decrease in renal function in determining does.

Side Effects

- **CNS:** Dizziness, headache and seizures
- **GI:** Hepatotoxicity, abdominal discomfort, diarrhea, nausea and vomiting
- **Dermatology: Exofoliative skin disorders including systemic -Johnson syndrome. Endo:** Hypocalemia, hypertriglyceridemia
- **Miscellaneous:** Allergic reaction including anaphylaxis.

Nursing Assessment and Management

Assess infected area and mentioned CSF culture before and periodically during therapy.

- Specimens for culture should be taken before instituting therapy. Therapy may be stated before result are obtained
- Monitored liver function tests before and periodically during therapy may cause increased aspartate aminotransferase (AST), alanine aminotransferase (ALT), serum alkaline phosphate and bilirubin.

NIFEDIPINE

Classification

- **Therapeutics:** Antianginal, antihypertensive
- **Pharmacologic:** Calcium channel blockers
- Pregnancy Category C

Action

Inhibits calcium transport into myocardial and vascular smooth muscle cells, resulting in inhibition of excitation-contraction coupling and subsequent contraction.

Therapeutic effects: Systematic vasodilatation, resulting in decreased blood pressure. Coronary vasodilatation, resulting in decreased frequency and severity of attacks of angina.

Indication

Management of hypertension, angina pectoris, vasopastic angina. Unlabeled Use: Prevention of migraine headache. Management of congestive heart failure (CHF) or cardiomyopathy.

Suppression of threatened or established preterm labor before 34 weeks gestation, where this is not contraindicated.

Contraindication

Contraindicated in hypersensitivity; sick sinus syndrome; 2nd–3rd degree AV block. Geri: Short acting forms appear on beers lished due to increased risk of hypotension and constipation.

Adverse Effect

- **CNS:** Headache, abnormal dreams, anxiety, confusion, dizziness and drowsiness
- **EENT:** Blurred vision, disturbed equilibrium, epistaxsis, tinnitus
- **Respiratory:** Cough, dyspnea, shortness of breath
- **CVS:** Arrhythmias, CHF Chest pain
- **GI:** Incresed liver function test.

Interaction

- **Drug–drug:** Addictive hypotension may occur when used concurrently with fentanyl, other hypertensive, nitrates
- **Drug–food:** Grapefruit and grape fruit juice increased serum level and effect.

Routes and Dosages

Adult: 10–30 mg 3 times daily or 10–20 mg twice daily as immediate or 30–90 mg once daily as sustained release. (PO)

Nursing Assessment and Management

- Monitor blood pressure and pulse before therapy, during dose titration and periodically during therapy. Monitor ECG periodically during prolonged therapy
- Monitor intake and output ratios and daily weight. Assess the sign of CHF
- **Geri:** Assess fall risk and institute fall prevention strategies
- Monitor hepatic and renal function periodically during long-term therapy.

Nursing Process Focus

Patients Receiving Nifedipine

Assessment

- **Prior to administration:**
  - Obtain complete health history including possible drug interactions and allergies
  - Obtain ECG and vital signs, including blood pressure
  - Assess neurological status and level of consciousness
  - Auscultate chest sounds for rales or rhonchi ("crackles") indicative of pulmonary edema
  - Assess lower limbs for edema.
- **Potential Nursing Diagnoses**
  - Ineffective health Maintenance, related to disease process
  - Deficient knowledge, related to drug action and side effects
  - Decreased cardiac output, related to inadequate contractility
  - Ineffective tissue perfusion, related to decreased cardiac output.
- **Planning:** Patient goals and expected outcomes

The patient will:

  - Exhibit a reduction in systolic/diastolic blood pressure
  - Demonstrate understanding of the drug's action by accurately describing drug side effects and precautions
  - Demonstrate adequate tissue perfusion.
- **Interventions and (Rationales) Patient/Discharge Planning**
  - Monitor vital signs, especially blood pressure and heart rate. Monitor EKG during initial therapy. (Nifedipine dilates the main coronary arteries and arterioles, reducing blood pressure.)
  - Instruct the patient to monitor vital signs regularly, particularly blood pressure, ensuring proper use of home equipment
  - withhold medication for severe hypotensive readings as specified by the health care provider (e.g. "hold for levels below 80/50"). Immediately report palpitations or rapid heart beat
  - Observe for changes in level of consciousness, dizziness, fatigue, postural hypotension, increased chest pain (caused by vasodilation and/or hypotension
  - **Instruct the patient to** immediately report any change in consciousness, particularly sense of faintness, increase or return of chest pain or other angina like symptoms.

- **Instruct patient to:** Avoid abrupt changes in posture; rise slowly from prolonged periods of sitting/ lying down. Obtain blood pressure readings in sitting standing and supine positions to monitor fluctuations in blood pressure
- Monitor fluid and electrolyte balance
- Monitor for signs of congestive heart failure (CHF), an adverse reaction. (Edema is a sideeffect of nifedipine.)
- Instruct the patient to immediately report any severe shortness of breath, frothy sputum, profound fatigue and swelling which may be signs of heart failure or pulmonary edema.

METHYLDOPA

Classification
- **Therapeutic:** Antihypertensive
- **Pharmacological:** Antiadrenergic

Action
- **Stimulate CNS alpha:** Adrenergic receptor, producing a decreases in sympathetic outflow to heart, kidneys, and blood vessels. Result is decrease blood pressure and peripheral resistance, a slight decrease in heart rate, and no change in cardiac output
- **Therapeutic effects:** Lowering of blood pressure.

Route and Dose
- **Adults:** 250–500 mg 2–3 times daily (PO)
- 250 mg 2–3 times daily and 500 mg –2g/day in 2–4 divided doses; maximum 3g/day (IV)
- **Children:** 10 mg/kg/day (PO)
- 5–10 mg/kg in divided doses; maximum 65 mg/kg or 3g daily. (IV)

Indication
Management of moderate to severe hypertension.

Contraindication
- Active hepatic disease
- History of methyldopa-associated liver dysfunction
- Concomitant monoamine oxidase inhibitors.

Side Effects
- **CNS:** Sedation, headache, asthenia
- **CVS:** Orthostatic hypotension, bradycardia and edema
- **GI:** GI upset, dry mouth, diarrhea
- **Dermatology:** Rash
- **EENT:** Nasal congestion
- **Hepatic:** Liver dysfunction
- **Hematology:** Hemolytic anemia.

Nursing Assessment and Management

- Monitor blood pressure and pulse frequently during initial dose adjustment and periodically during therapy
- Monitor frequency of prescription refills to determine compliance
- Monitor intake and output ratios and weight assess for edema daily, especially at beginning of therapy. Report weight gain or edema; sodium and water retention may be treated with diuretic
- Assess patient for depression or other alteration of mental status
- Monitor temperature during therapy
- **Lab test:** Monitor renal and hepatic function and CBC before and periodically during therapy
- Do not confuse methyldopa with levodopa or L-dopa
- Shake suspension before administration.

MAGNESIUM SULFATE

Classifications

Therapeutic: Mineral and electrolyte replacements/supplements.

Action

- Essential for the activity of many enzymes
- Plays an important role in neurotransmission and muscular excitability.

Therapeutic effects

- Replacements in deficiency states
- Resolution of eclampsia.

Routes and Dosages

Treatment of deficiency (expressed as mg of Magnesium)

- **Adults:** Severe deficiency –250 mg/kg over 4 hr; mild deficiency –1 g q 6 hr for 4 doses. (IM)
- **Adults:** Severe deficiency –5 g. (IV)

Eclampsia/Pre-eclampsia

- **Adults:** 4–5 g by IV infusion, concurrently with up to 5 g IM in each buttock; then 4–5 g IM 4hr or 4g by IV
- Infusion followed by 1–2 g/hr continuous infusion (not to exceed 40g/day or 20g/48hr in the presence of severe renal insufficient.

Part of Parenteral Nutrition

- **Adults:** 4–24g/mEq. (IV)
- **Children:** 0.25—0.5mEq/kg/day. (IV)

Indications

- Treatment/prevention of hypermagnesemia
- Convulsion in severe eclampsia or preeclampsia. Unlabelled uses:
  - Preterm labor
  - Treatment of torsades de pointes.

Contraindications and Precautions

Contraindicated in the following cases

- Hypermagnesemia
- Hyperpocalcemia
- Anuria
- Heart block
- Active labor or within 2 hours of delivery (unless- used for preterm labor).

Use Cautiously in:

- Any degree of renal insufficiency.

Side Effects

- **CNS:** Drowsiness
- **Respiratory:** Decreased respiratory rate
- **CV:** Arrhythmias, bradycardia, hypotension
- **GI:** Diarrhea
- **Derma:** Flushing and sweating
- **Metab:** Hypothermia.

Nursing Assessment and Management

- **Hypomagnesemia/Anticonvulsant:** Monitor pulse, blood pressure, respirations, and ECG frequently throughout administration of parenteral magnesium sulfate. Respirations should be at least 16 min before each dose.
- Monitor neurologic status before and throughout therapy; institute seizure precautions. Patellar reflex (knee jerk) should be tested before each parenteral dose of magnesium sulfate. If response is absent, no additional doses should be administered is obtained.
- Monitor newborn for hypotension, hyporeflexia, and respiratory depression if mother has received magnesium sulfate.
- Monitor intake and out ratios. Urine output should be maintained at a level of at least 100 mL/4hr.

RANTAC

Classification

- **Therapeutic:** Antiulcer agent
- **Pharmacologic:** Histamine H_2 antagonists

Action

- Inhibit the action of histamine at the H_2-receptor site located primarily in gastric parietal cell, resulting in inhibition of gastric acid secretion
- **Therapeutic effect:** Healing and prevention of ulcers decreased symptoms of gastroesophageal reflux. Decreased secretion of gastric acid.

Routes and Doses

- **Adult:** 150 mg 2 times daily or 300 mg once daily at bedtime (PO)
- 50 mg (2 mL) 6–8 hours. (IV, IM)

- **Children 1 month -16 years:** 2–4 mg/kg/day in divided doses (PO)
- 2–4 mg/kg/day divided doses 6–8 hours (IV, IM)
- **Neonates:** 2 mg/kg/day in divided doses (PO)
- 1.5 mg/kg/dose load, then in 12 hours start maintenance of 1.5-2 mg/kg/day divided dose in 12 hours. (IV)

Indications

Short-term treatment of active duodenal ulcer and benign gastric ulcer. Maintenance therapy for duodenal and gastric ulcer after healing of active ulcer. Management of GERD. Treatment of heartburn, acid indigestion.

Contraindication

- Hypersensitivity
- Renal impairment
- Phenylketonuria

Side Effects

- **CNS:** Confusion, dizziness, drowsiness, hallucination and headache
- **CVS:** Arrhythmias,
- **GI:** Constipation, diarrhea, drug induced hepatitis and nausea
- **Genitourinary system:** Erectile dysfunction,
- **Hematology:** Aplastic anemia, anemia, neutropenia and thrombocytopenia.

Nursing Assessment and Management

- Assess for epigastric or abdominal pain and frank or occult blood in the stool, emesis or gastric aspirate
- Assess geriatric and debilitated patients routinely for confusion
- **Lab test:** Monitor CBC with differential periodically during therapy
- Antagonize effect of penta gastrin and histamine during gastric acid secretion testing
- Administer with meal or immediately afterward and at bedtime to prolong effect
- Shake the oral suspension before administration.

ONDANSETRON

Classification

- **Therapeutic:** Anti-emetics
- **Pharmacologic:** 5-HT3 antagonists.

Action

- Blocks the effects of serotonin at 5-HT3 –receptor sites located in vagal nerve terminals and the chemoreceptor trigger zone in the CNS
- **Therapeutic effects:** Decreased incidence and severity of nausea and vomiting following chemotherapy or surgery.

Routes and Dosages

- **Adults and children>11 year:** *Prevention of chemotherapy induced nausea/vomiting*—**8 mg** 30 min prior to chemotherapy. (PO)
- *Prevention of radiation induced nausea/vomiting*—**8 mg** 1–2 hour prior to radiation; may be repeated for 8 hours depending on the type, location, extent of radiation
- *Prevention of post-operative nausea/vomiting*—**16 mg** 1 hour before induction of anesthesia
- **Children 4–11 year:** *Prevention of chemotherapy induced nausea/vomiting* –**4 mg** 30 min prior to chemotherapy and repeated 4 and 8 hour later. (PO)
- **Adults: 0.15 mg/kg** 15–30 min prior to chemotherapy, repeated 4–8 hour later. (IV)
- **Adults:** *Prevention of post-operative nausea/vomiting* –**4 mg** before induction of anesthesia
- **Children 6 months—18 year:** *Prevention of chemotherapy induced nausea/vomiting* –**0.15 mg/kg** 15–30 min before chemotherapy; repeated 4–8 hours later
- **Children 2–12 year and <40 kg:** *Prevention of post-operative nausea/vomiting*—**0.1 mg/kg.** (IV)
- **Children >40 kg:** *Prevention of post-operative nausea/vomiting*—**4 mg.** (IV)

Indications

Prevention of nausea and vomiting associated with chemotherapy and radiation therapy.

Contraindications

- **Hypersensitivity:** Orally disintegrating tablets contains aspartame and should not be used in patients with phenylketonuria.
- **Use cautiously in** liver impairment and abdominal surgery
- **Obstetric:** Lactation,
- **Pediatric:** Pregnancy and Lactation.

Side Effects

- **CNS:** Headache, dizziness, drowsiness, fatigue, weakness
- **GI:** Constipation, diarrhea, abdominal pain, dry mouth and increased liver enzymes
- **Neurology:** Extrapyramidal reactions.

Nursing Assessment and Management

- Assess patient for nausea, vomiting, abdominal distension, and bowel sounds prior to and following administration
- Assess patient for extrapyramidal effects periodically during therapy
- May cause increase in serum bilirubin, AST and ALT levels.

OMEPRAZOLE

Classification
- **Therapeutic:** Anti-Ulcer agent
- **Pharmacologic:** Proton-pump Inhibitor.

Action
Binds to an enzyme on gastric parietal cells in the presence of acidic gastric PH, preventing the final transport of hydrogen ions the gastric lumen.
- **Therapeutic Effects:** Diminished accumulation of acid in the gastric lumen with the lessened gastroesophageal reflux. Healing of duodenal ulcers.

Routes and Dosages
- **Adults:** H. pylori and duodenal ulcers—**40 mg** once morning daily for 2 weeks with clarithromycin, then **20 mg** once daily with clarithromycin **500 mg** for 2 weeks and amoxicillin **1,000 mg** for 10 days (PO)
- GERD—**20** mg once daily
- **Children 1–16 year and 5–9 kg:** GERD—**5 mg** once daily (PO)
- **Children 1–16 year and 10–19 kg:** GERD—**10 mg** once daily (PO)
- Children 1–16 year and >20 kg—GERD **20 mg** once daily. (PO)

Indications
GERD/maintenance of healing in erosive esophagitis. Short-term treatment of active benign gastric ulcer. Pathologic hypersecretory conditions, including Zollinger–Ellison syndrome. Reduction of risk of GI bleeding in critically ill patients.

Contraindications
- **Hypersensitivity:** Lactation-Discontinue omeprazole or discontinue breastfeeding.
- **Use cautiously in liver disease, Obstetric: Lactation, Pediatric:** Safely not established in pregnant of breastfeeding mother and children <1 year.

Side Effects
- **CNS:** Dizziness, drowsiness, fatigue, headache and weakness
- **CV:** Chest pain
- **GI:** Abdominal pain, acid regurgitation, constipation, diarrhea, nausea, vomiting
- **DERM:** Itching, rashes
- **MISC:** Allergic reactions.

Nursing Assessment and Management
- Assess patient routinely for epigastric or abdominal pain and frank or occult blood in the stool, emesis or gastric aspirate
- Monitor CBC with differential periodically during therapy

- May cause increase in AST and ALT, alkaline phosphatase, and bilirubin
- May cause serum gastrin concentrations to increase during first 1–2 week of therapy
- Monitor INR and prothrombin time in patients.

DULCOLAX

Classification

- **Therapeutic:** Laxatives
- **Pharmacologic:** Stimulant laxatives.

Action

Stimulates peristalsis. Alters fluid and electrolyte transport, producing fluid accumulation in the colon. Therapeutic effects: Evacuation of the colon.

Indications

Treatment of constipation. Evacuation of the bowel before radiologic studies or surgery. Part of a bowel regimen in spinal cord injury patients.

Contraindications/Precautions

Contraindicated in hypersensitivity, abdominal pain, obstruction, nausea or vomiting (especially with fever or other signs of an acute abdomen).

Adverse Reactions/Side Effects

GI: Abdominal cramps, nausea, diarrhea and rectal burning
F and E: Hypokalemia (with chronic use)
Musculoskeletal: Muscle weakness (with chronic use)
Miscellaneous: Protein-losing enteropathy, tetany (with chronic use).

Route/Dosage

- **Adults and Children -12 years:** 5- 15 mg/day (up to 30 mg/day) as a single dose. (PO)
- **Children 3–11 years:** 5–10 mg/day (0.3 mg/kg) as a single dose. (PO)

Nursing Assessment and Management

- Assess patient for abdominal distention, presence of bowel sounds, and usual pattern of bowel function.
- Assess color and consistency, and amount of stool produced.

Implementation

- Do not confuse Dulcolax (bisacodyl) with Dulcolax (docusate sodium)
- May be administered at bedtime for morning results
- **PO:** Taking on an empty stomach will produce more rapid results
- Do not crush or chew enteric-coated tablets. Take with a full glass of water or juice

- Do not administer oral doses within 1 hr of milk or antacids; this may lead to premature dissolution of tablet and gastric or duodenal irritation
- Advise patients, other than those with spinal cord injuries, that laxatives should be used only for short-term therapy. Prolonged therapy may cause electrolyte imbalance and dependence
- Advise patient to increase fluid intake to at least 1,500–2,000 mL/day during therapy to prevent dehydration
- Encourage patients to use other forms of bowel regulation (increasing bulk in the diet, increasing fluid intake or increasing mobility). Normal bowel habits may vary from 3 times/day to 3 times/wk.
- Instruct patients with cardiac disease to avoid straining during bowel movements (Valsalva maneuver)
- Advise patient that bisacodyl should not be used when constipation is accompanied by abdominal pain, fever, nausea, or vomiting.

LASIX

Classification

- **Therapeutic:** Diuretics
- **Pharmacologic:** Loop diuretics

Action

Inhibits the reabsorption of sodium and chloride from the loop of Henle and distal renal tubule. Increases renal excretion of water, sodium, chloride, magnesium, potassium, and calcium. Effectiveness persists in impaired renal function.

Therapeutic effects: Diuresis and subsequent mobilization of excess fluid (edema and pleural effusions). Decreased BP.

Routes and Dosages

- Edema
- **Adults:** 20–80 mg/day as a single dose initially (PO)
- **Adults:** 20–40 mg (IM, IV)

Indications

- Edema due to heart failure, hepatic impairment or renal disease
- Hypertension.

Contraindications/Precautions

Contraindicated in hypersensitivity, cross-sensitivity with thiazides and sulfonamide may occur, hepatic coma or anuria, some liquid products may contain alcohol, avoid in patients with alcohol intolerance.

Adverse Reactions/Side Effects

- **CNS:** Blurred vision, dizziness, headache and vertigo
- **EENT:** Hearing loss and tinnitus
- **CVS:** Hypotension

- **GI:** Anorexia, constipation, diarrhea, dry mouth, dyspepsia, liver enzymes, nausea, pancreatitis and vomiting
- **GU:** Excessive urination, nephrocalcinosis
- **Dermatology:** Erythema multiforme, stevens-johnson syndrome, toxic epidermal Necrolysis, photosensitivity, pruritis, rash, urticaria.
- **Endocrinology:** Hypercholesterolemia, hyperglycemia, hypertriglyceridemia, hypercupremia.

Nursing Assessment and Management

Assessment

- Assess fluid status. Monitor daily weight, intake and output ratios, amount and location of edema, lung sounds, skin turgor and mucous membranes. Notify health care professional if thirst, dry mouth, lethargy, weakness, hypotension or oliguria occurs
- Monitor BP and pulse before and during administration. Monitor frequency of prescription refills to determine compliance in patients treated for hypertension
- **Gesiatric:** Diuretic use is associated with increased risk for falls in older adults. Assess falls risk and implement fall prevention strategies
- Assess patients receiving digoxin for anorexia, nausea, vomiting, muscle cramps, paresthesia, and confusion. Patients taking digoxin are at increased risk of digoxin toxicity because of the potassium-depleting effect of the diuretic. Potassium supplement or potassium-sparing diuretics may be used concurrently to prevent hypocalcemia
- Assess patient for tinnitus and hearing loss. Audiometry is recommended for patient receiving prolonged high-dose IV therapy. Hearing loss is most common after rapid or high-dose IV administration in patients with decreased renal function or those taking other ototoxic drug
- Assess for allergy to sulfonamides
- Assess patient for skin rash frequently during therapy. Discontinue furosemide at first sign of rash; may be life-threatening. Stevens-Johnson syndrome, toxic epidermal necrolysis, or erythema multiforme may develop. Treat symptomatically may recur once treatment is stopped.

Implementation

- Do not confuse Lasix with Luvox
- If administering twice daily, give last dose no later than 5 pm to minimize disruption of sleep cycle
- IV route is preferred over IM route for parenteral administration
- **PO:** May be taken with food or milk to minimize gastric irritation. Tablets may be crushed if patient has difficulty in swallowing
- Do not administer discolored solution or tablets
- Instruct patient to take furosemide as directed. Take missed doses as soon as possible; do not double doses
- Caution patient to change positions slowly to minimize orthostatic hypotension. Caution patient that the use of alcohol, exercise during hot weather, or standing for long periods during therapy may enhance orthostatic hypotension
- Instruct patient to consult health care professional regarding a diet high in potassium
- Advise patient to contact health care professional of weight gain more than 3 lbs in 1 day
- Instruct patient to notify health care professional of all medicine or over-the-counter medications, vitamins, or herbal products being taken and to consult health care professional before taking any OTC medications concurrently with this therapy

- Instruct patient to notify health care professional of medication regimen before treatment or surgery
- Caution patient to use sunscreen and protective clothing to prevent photosensitive-reactions
- Advise patient to contact health care professional immediately if rash, muscle weakness, cramps, nausea, dizziness, numbness, or tingling of extremities occurs.

INSULIN

Classification

- **Therapeutic:** Antidiabetics and hormones
- **Pharmacologic:** Pancreatics

Action

- **Lower blood glucose by** stimulating glucose uptake in skeletal muscle and fat, inhibiting hepatic glucose production
- **Other actions:** Inhibition of lipolysis and proteolysis, enhanced protein synthesis
- **Therapeutic effects:** Control of hyperglycemia in diabetic patients.

Routes and Dosages

- Dose depends on blood glucose, response, and many other factors.
- **Subcut (Adults and Children):** 0.5–1 unit/kg/day. Adolescents during rapid growth—0.8–1.2 units/kg/day.

Indications

Control of hyperglycemia in patients with type 1 or type 2 diabetes mellitus.

Contraindications/Precautions

- **Contraindicated in:** Hypoglycemia; Allergy or hypersensitivity to a particular type of insulin, preservatives or other additives.
- **Use cautiously in** stress and infection (may temporarily increase insulin requirements)
- Renal/hepatic impairment (may decrease insulin requirements)
- **Obstetric**: Pregnancy may temporarily increase insulin requirements
- **Pediatric:** Safety of Humalog not established.

Adverse Reactions/Side Effects

- **Endocrine:** Hypoglycemia
- **Local:** Erythema, lipodystrophy, pruritis and swelling
- **Miscellaneous:** Allergic reactions including anaphylaxis.

Nursing Assessment and Management

- Assess for symptoms of hypoglycemia (anxiety; restlessness; tingling in hands, feet, lips, or tongue; chills; cold sweats; confusion; cool, pale skin; difficulty in concentration; drowsiness; excessive hunger; headache; irritability; nightmares or trouble sleeping; nausea; nervousness; tachycardia; tremor; weakness; unsteady gait) and hyperglycemia (confusion, drowsiness; flushed, dry skin;

fruit-like breath odor; rapid, deep breathing, polyuria; loss of appetite; nausea; vomiting; unusual thirst) periodically during therapy.

- Monitor body weight periodically. Changes in weight may necessitate changes in insulin dose.
- **Lab test considerations:** May cause decrease serum inorganic phosphate, magnesium and potassium levels.
- Monitor blood glucose every 6 hour during therapy, more frequently in ketoacidosis and times of stress. A1C may also be monitored every 3–6 months to determine effectiveness.
- **Toxicity and overdose:** Overdose is manifested by symptoms of hypoglycemia. Mild hypoglycemia may be treated by ingestion of oral glucose. Severe hypoglycemia is a life-threatening emergency; treatment consists of IV glucose, glucagon, or epinephrine.

METFORMIN

Classification

- **Therapeutic:** Antidiabetics
- **Pharmacologic:** Biguanides

Action

Decreases hepatic glucose production. Decreases intestinal glucose absorption. Increases sensitivity to insulin
Therapeutic effects: Maintenance of blood glucose.

Routes and Doses

- **Adults and children > 17 years:** 500 mg twice daily; may increase by 500 mg at weekly intervals up to 2000 mg/day. (PO)
- **Children > 10 years:** 500 mg twice daily, may be increased by 500 mg/day at 1 week intervals, up to 2000 mg/day in 2 divided doses. (PO)

Indications

Management of type 2 diabetes mellitus; may be used with diet, insulin, or sulfonylurea oral hypogly-cemic.

Contraindications

Hypersensitivity, metabolic acidosis; dehydration, sepsis, hypoxemia, hepatic impairment, excessive alcohol use (acute or chronic); renal dysfunction; radiographic studies requiring IV iodinated contrast media.

- **Use cautiously in** concurrent renal disease
- **Geriatrics:** Geriatric/debilitated patients
- **Chronic alcohol use:** Serious medical conditions (MI, Stroke); Patients undergoing stress.

Side Effects

- **GI:** Abdominal bloating, diarrhea, nausea, vomiting, unpleasant metallic taste
- **Endocrine:** Hypoglycemia
- **Fluid and electrolytes:** Lactic acidosis
- **Miscellaneous:** Decreased vitamin B12 levels.

Nursing Assessment and Management

Assessment

- When combined with oral sulfonylureas, observe for signs and symptoms of hypoglycemic reactions (abdominal pain, sweating, hunger, weakness, dizziness, headache, tremor, tachycardia and anxiety)
- Patients who have been well controlled on metformin who develop illness or laboratory abnormalities should be assessed for ketoacidosis or lactic acidosis
- Monitor serum glucose and glycosylated hemoglobin periodically during therapy to evaluate effectiveness of therapy
- Assess renal functions before initiating and at least during therapy. Discontinue metformin, if renal impairment occurs.

Potential Nursing Diagnosis

- **Imbalanced nutrition:** More than body requirements
- Noncompliance

Implementation

- Patients stabilized on a diabetic regimen who are exposed to stress, fever, trauma, infection or surgery may require administration of insulin. Withhold metformin and reinstitute after resolution of acute episode.
- Metformin therapy should be temporarily discontinued by patients requiring surgery involving restricted foods and fluid. Resume metformin when oral intake has resumed and renal function is normal.
- Withhold metformin before or at the time of studies requiring IV administration of iodinated contrast media and for 48 hour after study.

Patient and Family Teaching

- Instruct patient to take metformin at the same time each day, as directed. Take missed doses as soon as possible unless almost time for next dose. Do not double the doses
- Explain to patient that metformin helps to control hyperglycemia but does cure diabetes
- Encourage patient to follow prescribed diet, medication and exercise regimen to prevent hyperglycemic or hypoglycemic episodes
- Review signs of hypoglycemia and hyperglycemia with patients
- Instruct patient in proper testing of blood glucose and urine ketones
- Explain patient who are at risk of lactic acidosis and the potential need for discontinuation of metformin therapy.

ACETAMINOPHEN

Classification

- **Therapeutic:** Antipyretics, nonopioid analgesics
- **Pregnancy Category B**

Action

Inhibits the synthesis of prostaglandins that may serve as mediators of pain and fever, primarily in the CNS. Has no significant anti-inflammatory properties or GI toxicity.

- **Therapeutic effects:** Analgesia, Antipyretic.

Routes and Doses

- **Adults and children > 12 years:** 325–650 mg q 4–6 hr or 1 g 3–4 times daily or 1300 mg q 8 hr (not exceed 4 g or 2.5 g/24 hr in patient with hepatic and renal impairment. (PO)
- **Children 1–12 years:** 10–15 mg/kg/dose q 4–6 hr as needed. (not to exceed 5 doses/24 hrs). (PO)
- **Infants:** 10–15 mg/kg/doses q 4–6 hr as needed. (not to exceed 5 doses/24 hr). (PO)
- **Neonate:** 10–15 mg/kg/doses q 6–8 hr as needed. (PO)
- **Adult and children >12 years:** 325–650 mg q 4–6 hr as needed. (Rectal)
- Rectal (children 1 -12 years.

Indications

Mild pain and fever.

Contraindication

- Previous hypersensitivity, products containing alcohol, aspartame, saccharin, sugar, or tartrazine should be avoided in patient or intolerance to this compounds.
- **Use cautiously in** hepatic disease/renal diseases, chronic alcohol abuse and malnutrition.

Side Effects

- **GI:** Hepatic failure, hepatotoxicity
- **GU:** Renal failure
- **Hematology:** Neutropenia, pancytopenia, leucopenia
- **Dermatology:** Rash and urticaria
- **Pregnancy:** High doses can lead to attention deficit hypersensitivity disorder (ADHD), hyperkinetic disorder, asthma, cryptorchidism in children.

Nursing Assessment and Management

Assessment

- Assess overall health status and alcohol usage before administrating acetaminophen
- Assess amount, frequency and type of drug taken
- **Pain:** Assess type, location, and intensity prior to and 30–60 min following administration
- **Fever:** Assess fever, note presence of associated signs
- **Lab test considerations:** Evaluate hepatic, hematologic, and renal function
- **Toxicity and overdose:** If overdose occur, acetylcysteine is the antidote

Implementation

- Administer with full glass of water.

Patient and Family Teaching

- Advise patient to take medication as directed. Chronic excessive use of >4 g/day may lead to hepatotoxicity, renal or cardiac damage
- Advice patient to avoid alcohol (3 or more glasses per day increase the risk of liver damage)
- **Pediatric:** Advice patient or caregiver to check concentrations of liquid preparations. Demonstrate how to measure it using appropriate measuring device.

DICLOFENAC

Classification

Therapeutic: Nonopioid analgesics, nonsteroidal anti-inflammatory agents

Action

Inhibits prostaglandins synthesis.

- **Therapeutic effects:** Suppression of pain and inflammation. Relief of acute migraine attacks
- **Topical:** Clearance of actinic keratosis lesions.

Routes and Doses

Diclofenac Potassium

- **Adults:** Analgesic/antidysmenorrheal-100 mg initially, then 50 mg 3 times daily (PO)
- **Rheumatoid arthritis:** 50 mg 3–4 times daily, Osteoarthritis-50 mg 2–3 times daily.

Diclofenac sodium

- **Adults:** Rheumatoid arthritis-50 mg 3–4 times daily, Osteoarthritis-50 mg 2–3 times daily (PO)
- **Ankylosing spondylitis:** 25 mg 4 times daily, with an additional 25 mg given at bedtime.
- **Topical (Adult):**
  - **Solaraze:** Apply to lesions twice daily for 60-90 days; Voltaren gel – Lower extremities; Apply 4 g to affected area 4 times daily.

Indications

- **PO:** Management of inflammatory disorders including rheumatoid arthritis, osteoarthritis, ankylosing spondylitis primary dysmenorrhea. Relief of mild to moderate pain. Acute treatment of migraines (powder for oral solution)
- **Topical:** Management of actinic keratoses, osteoarthritis
- **Transdermal:** Acute pain due to minor strains, sprains and contusions.

Contraindications

Hypersensitivity to diclofenac or other components of formulation; Cross-sensitivity may occur with other NSAIDs including aspirin; Active GI bleeding/Ulcer disease; Patients undergoing coronary artery bypass graft surgery.

- **Use cautiously in:** Severe renal/hepatic disease, cardiovascular disease or risk factors for cardiovascular disease, heart failure, history of porphyria and History of peptic ulcer.
- **Pediatric:** Safety not established.
- **Geriatrics:** Dose reduction recommended; more susceptible to adverse reaction, including GI bleeding.
- **OB, Lactation:** Not recommended for use during second half of pregnancy.

Side Effects

- **CNS:** Dizziness and headache
- **EENT:** Tinnitus
- **CVS:** Hypertension
- **GI:** GI bleeding, abdominal pain, constipation, diarrhea, dyspepsia, flatulence, heartburn, nausea and vomiting
- **Genitourinary system:** Acute renal failure, hematuria
- **Dermatology:** Exfoliative dermatitis, Toxic epidermal necrolysis
- **Local:** Dry skin, exfoliation
- **Miscellaneous:** Allergic reactions including anaphylaxis.

Nursing Assessment and Management

Assessment

- Patients who have asthma, aspirin–induced allergy, and nasal polyps are at increased risk for developing hypersensitivity reactions
- Monitor blood pressure closely during initiation of treatment and periodically during therapy in patients with hypertension
- **Pain:** Assess pain and limitation of movements; note type, location, and intensity before and 30–60 minutes after administration
- **Arthritis:** Assess arthritic pain (note type, location and intensity) and limitation of movements during therapy
- **Actinic keratosis:** Assess lesions prior to and periodically during therapy
- Monitor CBC and liver function tests within 8 weeks of initiating diclofenac therapy
- Monitor blood urea nitrogen (BUN) and serum creatinine periodically during therapy
- **Dysmenorrhea:** Administer as soon as possible after the onset of menses. Prophylactic treatment has not been shown to be effective.

LIGNOCAINE

Classification

Therapeutic: Anesthetics (topical/local), Arrhythmics (class IB)

Action

- **IV, IM:** Suppresses automatic and spontaneous depolarization of the ventricles during diastole by altering the flux of sodium ions across cell membranes with little or no effect on heart rate
- **Local:** Produces local anesthesia by inhibiting transport of ions across neuronal membranes, thereby preventing initiation and conduction of normal nerve impulses
- **Therapeutic effects:** Control of ventricular arrhythmias, local anesthesia.

Routes and Doses

Ventricular tachycardia with a pulse or pulseless ventricular tachycardia, ventricular fibrillation

- **Adults:** 1–1.5 mg/kg bolus; may repeat doses of 0.5–0.75 mg/kg q 5–10 min up to a total dose of 3 mg/kg; may then start continuous infusion of 1–4 mg/min. (IV)

- **Adults:** Give 2–2.5 times the IV loading dose down the endotracheal tube, followed by a 10 mL saline flush. (Endotracheal)
- **Children:** 1 mg/kg bolus, followed by 20–50 mcg/kg/min continuous infusion; may administer second bolus of 0.5–1 mg/kg if delay between bolus and continuous infusion. (IV)
- **Children:** Give 2–3 mg/kg down the endotracheal tube followed by 5 mL saline flush. (Endotracheal)
- **Adults and Children ≥50 kg:** 300 mg; may be repeated in 60–90 minutes. (IM)

Local

- **Infiltration (Adults and Children):** Infiltrate affected area as needed
- **Topical (Adults):** Apply to affected area 23 times daily
- **Mucosal (Adults):** For anesthetizing oral surfaces-20 mg as 2 sprays/quadrant may be used. 15 mL of the viscous solution may be used q 3 hr for oral or pharyngeal pain. For anesthetizing the female urethra, 3–5 mL of the jelly or 20 mg as 2% solution may be used. For anesthetizing the male urethra, 5–10 mL of the jelly or 5–15 mL of 2% solution may be used before catheterization or 30 mL of jelly before cystoscopy or similar procedures. Topical solutions may be used to anesthetize mucous membranes of the larynx, trachea or esophagus
- **Patch (Adults):** Up to 3 patches may be applied once for up to 12 hours in any 24-hours period; consider smaller areas of application in geriatric or debilitated patients.

Availability

Autoinjector for IM injection: 300 mg/3 mL, *Direct IV injection:* 10 mg/mL (1%), 20 mg/mL (2%), *For IV admixture:* 100 mg/mL (10%), *Premixed solution for IV infusion:* 4 mg/mL (0.4%), 8 mg/mL (0.8%). *Injection for local infiltration/nerve block:* 0.5%, 1%, 2%, 4%, *In combination with: Epinephrine for local infiltration, Cream:* 4%, *Gel:* 0.5%, 2.5%", *Jelly:* 2%, *Liquid:* 5%, *Ointment:* 5%, *Transdermal system:* 5% patch, *Solution:* 4%, *Spray:* 10%, *Viscous solution:* 2%, *In combination with:* Prilocaine, with tetracaine, with bupivacaine with epinephrine.

Indications

- **IV:** Ventricular arrhythmias
- **IM:** Self-injected or when IV unavailable
- **Local:** Infiltration/mucosal/topical anesthetic
- **Patch:** Pain due to postherpetic neuralgia.

Contraindications

Hypersensitivity, cross-sensitivity may occur, third-degree heart block.

Use cautiously in liver disease, CHF, patients weighing <50 kg, and geriatric patients, respiratory depression, shock, heart block, Obstetric: Safety not established for lactation, Pediatric: Safety not established for transdermal patch.

Adverse Reactions/Side Effects

Applies mainly to systemic use.

- **CNS:** Seizures, confusion, drowsiness, blurred vision, dizziness, nervousness, slurred speech, tremor
- **EENT:** Mucosal use-decreased or absent gag reflex
- **CVS:** Cardiac arrest, arrhythmias, bradycardia, heart block, hypotension

- **GI:** Nausea, vomiting
- **Respiratory:** Bronchospasm
- **Local:** Stinging, burning contact dermatitis, erythema
- **Miscellaneous:** Allergic reactions, including anaphylaxis.

Nursing Assessment and Management

- **Antiarrhythmic:** Monitor ECG continuously and blood pressure and respiratory status frequently during administration
- **Anesthetic:** Assess degree of numbness of affected part
- **Transdermal:** Monitor for pain intensity in affected area periodically during therapy
- Serum electrolyte levels should be monitored periodically during prolonged therapy to prevent lignocaine toxicity and overdose. Therapeutic serum lignocaine levels range from 1.5 to 5 mcg/mL
- If symptoms of overdose or lignocaine toxicity (confusion, excitation, blurred or double vision, nausea, vomiting, ringing in ears, tremors, twitching, seizures, difficulty breathing, severe dizziness or fainting, and unusually slow heart rate) occur, stop infusion and monitor patient closely
- Advise patient to call for assistance during ambulation and transfer
- Advise patient to telephone health care professional immediately if symptoms of a heart attack occur
- Do not drive after administration unless absolutely necessary
- **Topical:** Apply Lignoderm patch to intact skin to cover the most painful area
- Do not drive after administration unless absolutely necessary
- **Topical:** Apply Lignoderm patch to intact skin to cover the most painful area.

PHENYTOIN

Classification

- **Therapeutic:** Antiarrhythmics (group IB), anticonvulsant
- **Pharmacologic:** Hydantoins.

Action

- Limits seizure propagation by altering ion transport. May also decrease synaptic transmission. antiarrhythmic properties as a results of shorting the action potential and decreasing automaticity
- **Therapeutic effect:** Diminished seizure activity. Termination of ventricular arrhythmias.

Routes and Doses

IM administration is not recommended due to erratic absorption and pain on injection.

Anticonvulsant

- **Adults:** Loading does of 15–20 mg/kg as extended capsule in divided dose is given every 2–4 hourly; maintenance does 5–6 mg/kg/day given in 1–3 divided does; usual dosing range = 200–1200 mg/day. (PO)
- **Children 10–16 years: 6–7 mg/kg/day in 2–3 divided dose (PO)**
- **Children 7–9 years:** 7–8 mg/kg/day in 2–3 divided does
- **Children 4–6 years:** 7.5–9 mg/kg/day in 2–3 divided does (PO)
- **Children 0.5– 3 years:** 8–10 mg/kg/day in 2–3 divided dose (PO)

- **Neonates up to 6 months:** 5–8 mg/kg/day in divided dose, may required q 8 hr dosing (PO)
- **Adult:** 15–20 mg/kg at 1–3 mg/kg/min. Maintenance does - same as PO dosing above (IV)
- **Children:** 15–20 mg /kg. (IV)

Antiarrhythmic

- **Adults:** 50–100 mg q 10– 15 min until arrhythmias is abolished or a total of 15 mg/kg has been given or toxicity occurs (IV)
- **Adult:** 250 mg QID for 1 day then 250 mg BID for 2 days then maintenance at 300 - 400 mg /day in divided does (PO)
- **Children:** 1.25 mg/kg q 5 min may repeat dose upto 15 mg/kg. Maintenance does 5– 10 mg/kg/day in 2–3 divided does IV or PO.

Indications

- Treatment/prevention of tonic-clonic (grand mal) seizure and complex partial seizure
- **Unlabeled use:** As an antiarrhythmic, particularly for ventricular arrhythmias associated with digoxin toxicity, prolonged QT interval, and surgical repair of congenital heart disease in children.
- Management of neuropathic pain, including trigeminal neuralgia.

Contraindications

- Hypersensitivity; hypersensitivity to propylene glycol (phenytoin injection only); alcohol intolerance (phenytoin injection and liquid only); sinus bradycardia, sinoatrial block, 2nd or 3rd degree heart block, or stokes adams syndrome (phenytoin injection only).
- **Use Cautiously in:** All patients hepatic or renal disease, patients with severe cardiac or respiratory diseases
- **OB:** Safety not established; may results in fetal hydantoin syndrome if used chronically or hemorrhage in the newborn if used at term; use with extreme caution
- **Lactation:** Safety not established
- **Pediatric:** Suspension contain sodium benzoate, metabolite of benzyl alcohol that can cause potentially fetal gasping syndrome in neonates
- **Geriatric:** Use of iv phenytoin may results in an increase risk of serious adverse reaction.

Side Effects

- **CNS:** Suicidal thought, ataxia, agitation, confusion, dizziness, drowsiness, dysarthria, dyskinesia, extrapyramidal syndrome, headache, insomnia, weakness
- **EENT:** Diplopia, nystagmus
- **CVS:** Hypotension, tachycardia
- **GI:** Gingival hyperplasia, nausea, constipation, drug-induced hepatitis, vomiting
- **Dermatology:** Hypertrichosis, rash, exfoliative dermatitis, pruritus, purple glove syndrome
- **Hematology:** Agranulocytosis, aplastic anemia, leukopenia, megaloblastic anemia and thrombocytopenia
- **Musculoskeletal:** Osteomalacia, osteoporosis.
- **Miscellaneous:** Allergic reaction including Stevens -Johnson syndrome, fever lymphadenopathy.

Nursing Assessment and Management

Assessment

- Monitored closely change in behavior that could indicate the emergence or worsening of suicidal thoughts or behavior or depression
- Assess oral hygiene. Various cleaning begins within 10 days of initiation of phenytoin therapy may help control gingival hyperplasia
- Assess patients for phenytoin hypersensitivity syndrome. Rash usually occurs within the first 2 weeks of therapy
- Observe patients for development of rash. Discontinue phenytoin at the first sign of skin reaction
- **Seizure:** Assess location, duration, frequency and characteristics of seizure activity. EEG may be monitored periodically throughout therapy
- Monitor blood pressure, ECG, and respiratory function continuously during administration of IV phenytoin and throughout period
- **Arrhythmias:** Monitored ECG continuously during treatment of arrhythmias
- May cause increase serum alkaline phosphatase, gamma glutamyl transferase and glucose levels
- Monitored serum folate concentrations periodically during prolonged therapy.

PENTAZOCINE

Classification

- **Therapeutic:** Opioid analgesics
- **Pharmacologic:** Opioid agonists/antagonists.

Action

- Binds to opiate receptors in the CNS. Alters perception of response to painful stimuli, while producing generalized CNS depression. Has partial antagonist properties, which may result in opioid withdrawal in physically dependent patients
- **Therapeutic effects:** Decrease in moderate to severe pain.

Routes and Dosages

- **PO (adults):** 50–100 mg q 3–4 hour (not to exceed 600 mg/day)
- **Subcut, IV, IM (Adults):** 30 mg q 3–4 hour. Obstetrical use – 20 mg IV or 30 mg IM when contractions become regular, may repeat q 2–3 hour for 2–3 doses.

Indications

Moderate to severe pain. Also used for: Analgesia during labor, sedation prior to surgery, Supplementation in balanced anesthesia.

Contraindications

- Hypersensitivity; patients who are physically dependent on opioids (may precipitate withdrawal)
- **Use cautiously in:** Head trauma, history of drug abuse, increased intracranial pressure, severe renal, hepatic or pulmonary disease, hypothyroidism, renal insufficiency, alcoholism.
- **Obstetric:** Has been during labor but may cause respiratory depression in newborn
- **Lactation:** Safety not established.

Side Effects

- **CNS:** Dizziness, euphoria, hallucinations, sedation, confusion, dysphoria and unusual dreams
- **EENT:** Blurred vision, miosis and diplopia
- **Resp:** Respiratory depression
- **CVS:** Hypertension, hypotension and palpitations
- **GI:** Nausea, constipation, dry, mouth, ileus and vomiting
- **GU:** Urinary retention.
- **Local:** Severe tissue damage at subcutaneous sites.

Nursing Assessment and Management

Assessment

- Assess type, location and intensity of pain prior to and 1 hour following PO, subcut or IM and 15–20 minutes following IV administration
- An equianalgesic chart should be used when changing routes or when changing from one opioid to another
- Assess blood pressure, pulse and respirations before and periodically during administration
- Assess prior analgesic history. Antagonistic properties may induce withdrawal symptoms (vomiting, restlessness, abdominal cramps, and increased blood pressure and temperature) in patients physically dependent on opioids
- Although, this drug has a low potential for dependence, prolonged use may lead to physical and psychological dependence and tolerance. This should not prevent patient from receiving adequate analgesia.

Implementation

- Accidental overdose of opioid analgesics has resulted to fatalities. Before administering, clarify all ambiguous orders, have second practitioner independently check original order and dose calculations
- Explain therapeutic value of medication prior to administration to enhance the analgesic effect
- Regularly administered doses may be more effective
- Co-administration with nonopioid analgesics may have addictive effects and may permit lower opioid doses
- Administer IM injections deep into well-developed muscle. Rotate sites of injections. Subcutaneous route may cause tissue damage with repeated injections.

Patient/Family Teaching

- Instruct patient on how and when to ask for pain medication
- Medication may cause drowsiness, dizziness, or hallucinations particularly in geriatric patients. Advice patient to call for assistance when ambulating. Institute fall prevention strategies
- Caution patient to change positions slowly to minimize orthostatic hypotension.

IRON SUCROSE

Classification

- **Therapeutic:** Antianemic
- **Pharmacologic:** Iron suplements

Action

An essential mineral found in hemoglobin, myoglobin, and many enzymes. Enters the blood stream and is transported to the reticuloendothelial system (liver, spleen, bone marrow), where it is separated out and becomes part of iron stores.

Therapeutic effects: Prevention and treatment of iron deficiency.

Routes and Doses

Adults (IV)

- **Hemodialysis dependent patient:** 100 mg (5 mL) during each dialysis section
- **Peritoneal dialysis dependent patient:** 300 mg (15 mL) infusion followed by another 300 mg (15 mL) infusion
- **Nondialysis dependent patient:** 200 mg (10 mL) on 5 different days within a 14 days.

Indications

Prevention and treatment of iron deficiency anemia, treatment of iron deficiency anemia in patients undergoing chronic hemodialysis and peritoneal dialysis, treatment of iron deficiency anemia in pregnancy.

Contraindications

Hemochromatosis, hemosiderosis or other evidence of iron overload; Anemias not due to iron deficiency; Some product contains alcohol, tartrazine or sulfites and should be avoided in patients with known intolerance or hypersensitivity.

Use cautiously in (PO): Peptic ulcer, ulcerative colitis, or regional enteritis, alcoholism, severe hepatic impairement, severe renal impairement, pre-existing cardiovascular disease, rheumatoid arthritis.

Obstetric, Lactation; - Pregnancy or lactation (safety of some parenteral products not established)

Side Effects

- **CNS:** IM, IV-seizures, dizziness, headache and syncope
- **RESP:** IV cough, dypnea
- **CV:** IM, IV – hypotention, hypertention and tachycardia
- **GI:** Nausea, PO, constipation, dark stools, diarrhea, epigastric pain, GI bleeding, IM, IV, taste disorder and vomiting
- **Dermatology:** IM, IV- flushing and urticaria
- **Local:** Pain at IM site and phlebitis (IV)
- **Miscellaneous:** Staining of teeth and allergic reactions.

Nursing Assessment and Management

Assessment

- Assess nutritional status and dietary history to determine possible cause of anemia and need for patient teaching
- Assess bowel function for constipation or diarrhea. Notify health care professional and use appropriate nursing measures should these occur

- **Iron dextran, iron sucrose, and sodium ferric gluconate complex:** Monitor blood pressure and heart rate frequently following IV administration until stable
- Assess patient for sign and symptoms of anaphylaxis (rash, pruritis, laryngeal edema, wheezing) Notify physician immediately if these occur
- Monitor hemoglobin, hematocrit, serum ferritin and transferrin saturation prior to and periodically during therapy
- Early symptoms of overdose includes stomach pain, fever, nausea, vomiting and diarrhea. Late symptoms include bluish lips, fingernails, and palms, drowsiness, weakness, tachycardia, etc.

IRON SORBITOL

Classification

- **Antianemic:** Ferrous fumarate, ferrous gluconate, ferrous sulfate, iron dextran, iron-polysaccharide, iron sorbitol, iron sucrose, sodium ferric gluconate
- **Nutritional supplement, mineral:** Ferrous fumarate, ferrous gluconate, ferrous sulfate, iron dextran, iron sorbitol and iron-polysaccharide

Action

Iron is an essential component in the physiological formation of hemoglobin, adequate amounts of which are necessary for effective erythropoiesis and the resultant oxygen transport capacity of the blood. A similar function is provided by iron in myoglobin production. Iron also serves as a cofactor of several essential enzymes, including cytochromes that are involved in electron transport. Iron is necessary for catecholamine metabolism and the proper functioning of neutrophils.

Routes and Dosages

- Adult and teenage males—10 milligrams (mg) per day
- Adult and teenage females—10 to 15 mg per day
- Pregnant females—30 mg per day
- Breastfeeding females—15 mg per day
- Children 7 to 10 years of age—10 mg per day
- Children 4 to 6 years of age—10 mg per day
- Children birth to 3 years of age—6 to 10 mg per day.

For Canada

- Adult and teenage males—8 to 10 mg per day
- Adult and teenage females—8 to 13 mg per day
- Pregnant females—17 to 22 mg per day
- Breastfeeding females—8 to 13 mg per day
- Children 7 to 10 years of age—8 to 10 mg per day
- Children 4 to 6 years of age—8 mg per day
- Children birth to 3 years of age—0.3 to 6 mg per day.

Indications

Jectofer injection is a medicine that is used for the treatment of iron deficiency anemia and other conditions.

The complete list of uses and indications for Jectofer Injection is as follows:

- Iron deficiency anemia
- Jectofer injection may also be used for purposes not listed here.

Contraindications

Hypersensitivity to Jectofer injection is a contraindication. In addition, Jectofer Injection should not be used if you have the following conditions:

- Allergic reactions
- Iron overload
- Megaloblastic anemia due to vitamin B12 deficiency
- Repeated blood transfusion.

Adverse Effects

Tachycardia, restlessness, gastrointestinal irritation, convulsions, hypotension collapse, nausea, metabolic acidosis, abdominal pain, vomiting, drowsiness, heartburn, hemorrhagic gastroenteritis, constipation and diarrhea.

Nursing Assessment and Management

- Assess nutritional status and dietary history to determine possible cause of anemia and need for patient teaching
- Assess bowel function for constipation or diarrhea. Notify health care professional and use appropriate nursing measures should these occur.
- **Lab test considerations:** Monitor hemoglobin, hematocrit, and reticulocyte values prior to and every 3 wk during the first 2 months of therapy and periodically thereafter. Serum ferritin and iron levels may also be monitored to assess effectiveness of therapy
- Occult blood in stools may be obscured by black coloration of iron in stool. Guaiac test results may occasionally be false-positive. Benzidine test results are not affected by iron preparations.
- **Toxicity and overdose:** Early symptoms of overdose include stomach pain, fever, nausea, vomiting (may contain blood), and diarrhea. Late symptoms include bluish lips, fingernails, and palms; drowsiness; weakness; tachycardia; seizures; metabolic acidosis; hepatic injury; and cardiovascular collapse. Patient may appear to recover prior to the onset of late symptoms. Therefore, hospitalization continues for 24 hr after patient becomes asymptomatic to monitor for delayed onset of shock or GI bleeding. Late complications of overdose include intestinal obstruction, pyloric stenosis, and gastric scarring.
- If patient is comatose or seizing, gastric lavage with sodium bicarbonate is performed. Deferoxamine is the antidote. Additional supportive treatments to maintain fluid and electrolyte balance and correction of metabolic acidosis are also indicated

CALCIUM

Classification

- **Therapeutic:** Mineral and electrolyte replacement/supplement
- **Pharmacologic:** Antacids
- **Pregnancy Category C.**

Action

Essential for nervous, muscular, and skeletal systems. Maintain cell membrane and capillary permeability. Act as an activator in the transmission of nerve impulses and contraction of cardiac, skeletal, and smooth muscles. Essential for bone formulation and coagulation.

Therapeutic effects: Replacement of calcium in deficiency states.Control of hyperphosphatemia in end stage renal diseases.

Routes and Doses

- **Adult:** 1–2 g/day (PO)
- **Children:** 45–65 mg/kg/day (PO)
- **Adults:** 7–14 mEq (IV)
- **Children:** 1–7 mEq (IV)

Indications

- Hypocalcemia, osteoporosis, hyperkalemia and hypermagnesemia and adjunct in cardiac arrest or calcium channel blocking agent toxicity
- **Calcium carbonate:** Use as antacid
- **Calcium acetate:** Control of hyperphosphatemia in end stage renal disease. In pregnancy to develop skeleton and heart in infant.

Contraindication

Hypercalcemia, renal calculi and ventricular fibrillation.

Use cautiously in: Patient receiving digitalis glycosides; severe respiratory insufficiency; renal diseases and cardiac disease.

Side Effects

- **CNS:** Syncope, tingling
- **CVS:** Cardiac arrest, arrythmias, bradycardia
- **GI:** Constipation, nausea vomiting
- **GU:** Calculi, hypercalciuria
- **Local:** Phlebitis.

Nursing Assessment and Management

Assessment

- Observe patient closely for symptoms of hypocalcemia (paresthesia, muscle twitching, laryngo-spasm, cardiac arrhythmias)

- Monitor blood pressure, pulse, ECG frequently throughout parental therapy
- Assess IV site for patency. Extravasations may cause cellulites, necrosis and sloughing.

Implementation

- **High alert:** Errors with calcium gluconate and chloride have occurred secondary to confusion
- **PO:** Administer calcium carbonate or phosphate 1–1.5 hours after meals and at bedtime
- **IM:** IM administration may cause necrosis and tissue sloughing. Do not administer IM
- **IV:** Administer slowly. High concentration may cause cardiac arrest.

Patient/family teaching

- Advice patient that calcium may cause constipation. Review methods of preventing constipation (increase bulk in diet fluid intake and increasing mobility)
- Encourage client to include milk, dairy products soya milk, cereals, yogurt cheese almonds and green leafy vegetables
- Advise to inform health team if brittle nails, aching muscle, weak bones, muscle cramps which is the sign of calcium deficiency in pregnancy.

FOLIC ACID

Classification

- **Theraputic:** Antianemics, vitamins
- **Pharmacological:** Water-soluble vitamins.

Action

- Required for protein synthesis and red blood cell function. Stimulate the production of red blood cells, white blood cells and platelets
- Necessary for normal fetal development
- **Therapeutic effect:** Restoration and maintenance of normal hematopoiesis.

Routes and Doses

- **Adult and children > 11 years (IM, PO, IV):** 1 mg/day
- **Children >1 year (PO, IM, IV, Subcutaneous):** 1 mg/day
- **Infants (PO, IM, IV, Subcutaneous):** 15 mcg/kg/day.

Indications

Prevention and treatment of megaloblastic and macrocytic anemias
Given during pregnancy to promote normal fetal development.

Contraindication

Contraindicated in

- Uncorrected pernicious, aplastic or normocytic anemias
- **Pediatric:** Preparation containing benzyl alcohol should not be used in newborns.

Use cautiously in

- Undiagnosed anemias.

Side Effects

- **Dermatology:** Rash,
- **CNS:** Irritability, difficulty sleeping, malaise and confusion
- **Miscellaneous:** Fever.

Nursing Assessment and Management

Assessment

- Assess the patient for signs of megaloblastic anemia (fatigue, weakness and dyspnea) before and periodically throughout therapy
- **Lab test consideration:** Monitor plasma folic acid levels, hemoglobin, hematocrit and reticulocyte count before and periodically during therapy
- May cause decrease serum concentration of other B complex vitamins when given in high continuous doses.

Implementation

- Do not confuse folic acid with folinic acid
- Because of infrequency of solitary vitamin deficiencies, combinations are commonly administrate
- **PO:** Antacid should be given at least 2 hr after folic acid
- **IV:** Solution ranges from yellow to orange yellow in color
- **IV administration:**
  - **Direct IV (Diluent):** Dilute with dextrose or 0.9 % NaCl
  - **Concentration:** 0.1 mg/mL
  - **Rate:** 5 mg/min.

  Continuous infusion: May be added to hyperalimentation solution.

Family Teaching

- Encourage patient to comply with diet recommendation of health care professional
- Explain that the best source of vitamins is a well balanced diet with foods from the four basic food groups
- Folic acid in early pregnancy is necessary to prevent neural tube defect
- Foods high in folic acid include vegetables, fruits and organ meats; heat destroys folic acid in foods
- Explain the folic acid make urine more intensely yellow
- Emphasis the importance of follow–up exams to evaluate progress.

PYRIDOXINE

Classification

- **Therapeutic:** Vitamins
- **Pharmacologic:** Water-soluble vitamins

Action

- Required for amino acids, carbohydrate, and lipid metabolism. Used in the transport of amino acid, formation of neurotransmitters, and synthesis of heme.
- **Therapeutic effects:** Prevention of pyridoxine deficiency. Prevention or reversal of neuropathy associated with hydralazine, penicillamine or isoniazid therapy.

Routes and Dosages

Prevention of deficiency (recommended daily allowance)

- **Adults and children >14 years:** PO, 1.2 -1.7 mg/day (larger does required with cycloserine, ethionamide, hydralazine, immunosuppressants, isoniazid penicillamine, and estrogen-containing oral contraceptives)
- **Children 9–13 years:** PO 1 mg/day
- **Children 1–8 years:** PO 0.5–0.6 mg/day.

Treatment of Deficiency

- **Adults:** PO, 2.5–10 mg/day until clinical signs are corrected, then 2–5 mg/day
- **Children:** PO, 5–25 mg/day for 3 weeks, then 1.5–2.5 mg/day.

Pyridoxine-dependent Seizures

Neonates and infants: PO, IM, IV, 10– 100 mg initially then 50–100 mg/day orally

Drug-Induced Neuritis

Adults: PO, Treatment-100–300 mg/day; prophylaxis-25–100 mg/day.

Isoniazid Overdose (>10g)

Adults and children: IM, IV Amount in mg equal to amount of isoniazid ingested given as 1–4 g IV, then 1 g 1M q 30 min.

Indications

Treatment and prevention of pyridoxine deficiency (may be associated with poor nutritional status or chronic debilitating illnesses). Treatment of pyridoxine–dependent seizures in infants. Treatment and prevention of neuropathy, which may develop from isoniazid, penicillamine or hydralazine therapy. Management of isoniazid overdose>10 g.

Contraindications/Precautions

Hypersensitivity to pyridoxine or any component

Use cautiously in: Parkinson's disease (treatment with levodopa only); OB chronic ingestion of large doses may produce pyridoxine – dependency syndrome in newborn.

Adverse Reactions/Side Effects

Adverse reaction listed are seen with excessive doses only

- **Neurology:** Sensory neuropathy, paresthesia
- **Miscellaneous:** Pyridoxine-dependent syndrome.

Interactions

Drug-Drug interferes with the therapeutic response to Levodopa when use without carbidopa. Requirements are increased by isoniazid, hydralazine, chloramphenicol, penicillamine, estrogens, and immunosuppressants. Decreases serum level of phenobarbital and phenytoin.

Nursing Assessment and Management

Assessment

- Assess patient for signs of vitamin B6 deficiency[anemia, dermatitis, irritability, seizures, nausea, and vomiting] before and periodically throughout therapy
- Protect parental solution from light, decomposition will occur.

Management

- **PO:** Extended release capsules and tablets should be swallowed whole, without crushing, breaking and chewing
- **IM:** Rotates sites, churning or stringing at site may occur
- **IV:** May be administered slowly by direct IV or as fusion in standard IV solution.monitor respiratory rate, heart rate and blood pressure when administrating large IV doses
- **Rate:** Infuse rate of 15–30 minutes and up to 3 hours has been used
- **Additive incompatibility:** Alkaline solution, riboflavin
- Explain that the best source of vitamins is the well balanced diet with food from the four basic food groups. Food high in vitamin B6 include bananas, whole grain cereals, potatoes, lima beans and meats
- Patient self-medicating with vitamins supplements should be cautioned not to exceed RDA
- Emphasize the importance of follow up exams to evaluate progress.

MIFEPRISTONE

Classification

- **Therapeutic:** Abortifacients
- **Pharmacologic:** Antiprogestational agents.

Action

Antagonize endometrial and myometrial effects of progesterone. Sensitize the myometrium to contraction-inducing activity of prostaglandins.
Theraputic Effect: Termination of pregnancy.

Routes and Dosages

Adult: PO, 600 mg (given as 200 mg tablet) as a single dose, followed on

Day 3–400 mcg misoprostol, unless abortion as occurred and has been confirmed byclicnical or ultrasonic examination.

Indication

Medical termination of intrauterine pregnancy up to day 49 of pregnancy.

Contraindication

Presence of IUD, confirmed or suspected ectopic pregnancy, undiagnosed adnexal mass, Chronic adrenal failure, Concurrent long-term corticosteroids therapy, bleeding disorder or concurrent anticongulant therapy and inherited porphyrias.

Use cautiously in: Chronic medical conditions such as cardiovascular, hypertensive, hepatic, renal, or respiratory disease.

Women >35 years old or who smoke >10 cigarette/day.

Side Effects

- **CNS:** Dizziness, fainting, headache, weakness
- **GI:** Abdominal pain, diarrhea, nausea, vomiting
- **GU:** Uterine bleeding, uterine cramping, ruptured ectopic pregnancy and pelvic pain.

Nursing Assessment and Management

- Determine duration of pregnancy. Pregnancy is dated from the first day of the menstrual period in a presumed 238 days cycle with ovulation occurring at mid-cycle and can be determined by menstrual history and clinical examination
- Asses the amount of bleeding and cramping during treatment
- Any IUD should be removed prior to mifepristone administration
- **PO:** On day 1, after the patient has read the medication guide and signed the patient agreement, administer three 200 mg tablet of mifepristone as a single dose
- On day 3 unless abortion has occurred and been confirmed by clinical examination or ultrasound, administer two 200 mcg tablet of misoprostol
- On day14, confirm the termination of pregnancy which is by clinical examination
- Advise patient of treatment and its effects
- Inform the patient that vaginal bleeding and uterine cramping will probably occur and prolonged long and heavy bleeding is not proof of complete expulsion. Bleeding or spotting occur for an average of 9–16 days; but may continue for 30 days
- Advise patient that if the treatment fails, there is a risk of fetal malformation; medical abortion failure are managed by surgical termination
- Caution patient to notify health care professional immediately if she develops weakness, nausea, vomiting, diarrhea, with or without abdominal pain or fever more than 24 hours after taking mifepristone; may indicate life-threating sepsis
- Instruct patient in a step to take in an emergency situation, including precise instruction and a telephone number to call if has any problem
- Caution patient that pregnancy can occur following termination of pregnancy and before resumption of normal menses. contraception can be initiated as soon as pregnancy termination is confirmed, or before sexual intercourse is resumed.

CARBOPROST

Classification

- **Therapeutic:** Abortifacients
- **Pharmacologic:** Oxytocics, prostaglandins
- **Pregnancy Category C.**

Indications

Induction of mid-trimester abortion. Treatment of postpartum hemorrhage that has not responded to conventional therapy.

Action

Causes uterine contractions by directly stimulating the myometrium.
Therapeutic effects: Expulsion of fetus. Control of postpartum bleeding.

Pharmacokinetics

- **Absorption:** Well absorbed following IM administration
- **Distribution:** Unknown
- **Metabolism and Excretion:** Unknown
- **Half-life:** Unknown.

Time/Action Profile (peak noted as mean abortion time)

Route onset peak duration

IM unknown 16 hr unknown

Contraindications/Precautions

- **Contraindicated in:** Hypersensitivity, acute pelvic inflammatory disease, active pulmonary, renal, or hepatic disease
- **Use Cautiously in:** Uterine scarring, asthma, hypotension, hypertension, cardiac disease, adrenal disease, anemia, jaundice, diabetesmellitus and epilepsy.

Adverse Reactions/Side Effects

- **CNS: Dizziness, headache**
- **Resp: Wheezing**
- **GI:** Diarrhea, nausea, vomiting, abdominal **pain, cramps**
- **GU: Uterine rupture**
- **Dermatology: Flushing. Misc:** Fever, chills, shivering.

Interactions

- **Drug-Drug:** Augments the effects of other **oxytocic agents**.
- **Route/Dosage**
- **Test Dose**
- **IM (Adults):** 100 mcg.
- **Abortifacient**
- **Adults:** IM, 250 mcg every 1.5–3.5 hr depending upon uterine response; may be increased to 500 mcg if several doses of 250 mcg produce inadequate response (not to exceed 2 days of continuous therapy or total dose of 12 mg)
- **Refractory Postpartum Uterine Bleeding**
- **Adults:** IM, 250 mcg; may be repeated every 15–90 min (total dose not to exceed 2 mg).

Nursing Assessment and Management

Assessment

- Monitor frequency, duration, and force of contractions and uterine resting tone

- Notify physician or other health care professional if contractions are absent or last more than 1 min
- Monitor temperature, pulse and BP periodically throughout course of therapy
- Large dose may cause hypertension. Temperature elevation beginning 1 to 16 hours after initiation of therapy and lasting for several hours is not unusual
- Auscultate breath sounds. Wheezing and sensation of chest tightness may indicate hypersensitivity reaction
- Assess for nausea, vomiting, and diarrhea. Vomiting and diarrhea occur in approximately two-thirds of patients. Premedication with antiemetic and antidiarrheal is recommended
- Monitor amount and type of vaginal discharge. Notify physician or other health care professional immediately if symptoms of hemorrhage (increased bleeding, hypotension, pallor, tachycardia) occur.

Potential Nursing Diagnoses

Deficient knowledge, related to medication regimen (Patient/Family Teaching)

Implementation

- Avoid contact with skin. Wash skin thoroughly immediately after spillage
- Opioid analgesic may be given for uterine cramping
- 2015 F.A. Davis Company **2**
- Store in refrigerator.
- **IM:** Administer deep IM. Dose may be repeated every 1.5–3.5 hours. Rotate sites.

Patient/Family Teaching

- Explain purpose of vaginal examinations (to assess for trauma to cervix)
- Instruct patient to notify health care professional immediately if fever and chills, foul-smelling vaginal discharge, lower abdominal pain, or increased bleeding occurs.

Evaluation/Desired Outcomes

- Complete abortion
- Control of postpartumor postabortal hemorrhage.

PROGESTERONE

Classification

- **Therapeutic:** Hormones
- **Pharmacologic:** Progestins.

Action

- **Produces:** Secretory changes in the endometrium, increases in basal body temperature, histologic changes in vaginal epithelium, relaxation of uterine smooth muscle, mammary alveolar tissue growth, pituitary inhibition, Withdrawal bleeding in the presence of estrogen.
- **Therapeutic effects:** Restoration of hormonal balance with control of uterine bleeding. Successful outcome in assisted reproduction.

Route and Dose

- **Adults:** PO, Secondary amenorrhea - 400 mg once daily for 10 days; prevention of postmenopausal estrogen-induced endometrial hyperplasia-200 mg once daily for 14 days.
- **Vag (Adults):** Secondary amenorrhea-45 mg once every other day for up to 6 doses. Corpus luteum insufficiency or assisted reproduction technology- For luteal support: 90 mg; for in vitro fertilization: 90 mg; Partial or complete ovarian failure –90 mg.
- **Children> 6 month:** IM, Secondary amenorrhea- 100–150 mg for 6–8 days. Dysfunctional uterine bleeding-5–10 mg daily for 6 days. Corpus luteum insufficiency –12.5 mg/day at onset of ovulation for 2 weeks.

Indications

Secondary amenorrhea and abnormal uterine bleeding due to hormonal imbalance.

- **Prometrium:** Prevention of cell over growth in the uterine lining in postmenopausal women who have not hysterectomy. Part of assisted reproductive technology in the management of infertility
- **Endometrium:** Support of embryo implantation and early pregnancy
- **Unlabeled Use:** Corpus luteum dysfunction.

Contraindications

- **Hypersensitivity:** Hypersensitivity to parabens or sesame oil, thromboembolic disease, cerebrovascular disease, severe liver disease, breast or genital cancer, porphyria, missed abortion
- **Obstetric:** Contraindicated except in corpus luteum dysfunction
- **Use cautiously in:** History of liver disease, renal disease, cardiovascular disease, seizure disorders, mental depression.

Side Effects

- **CNS:** Depression
- **EENT:** Renal thrombosis
- **CV:** Respiratory depression
- **CV:** Plumonary embolism, Thromboembolism
- **GI:** Gingival bleeding, hepatitis
- **GU:** Cervical erosions
- **Dermatology:** Chloasma, melasma, rashes
- **Endocrine:** Amenorrhea, breakthrough bleeding, breast tenderness, changes in menstrual flow, galactorrhoea, spotting
- **Local:** Irritation or pain (IM)
- **Miscellaneous:** Allergic reactions including Anaphylaxis, weight gain, weight loss.

Nursing Assessment and Management

Assessment

- Monitor blood pressure periodically during therapy
- Monitor intake and output ratios and weekly weight
- **Amenorrhea:** Assess patients usual menstrual history. Therapy should be discontinued if menses occur during therapy
- **Dysfunctional bleeding:** Monitor pattern and amount of vaginal bleeding.

Management

- **IM:** Shake vial before preparing IM dose. Administer deep IM. Rotate sites.
- **Vag:** Vaginal gel and insert are administered with disposable applicator provided by manufacturer. Ins
- Advice patient to report sign and symptoms of fluid retention (swelling of ankles and feet, weight gain), thromboembolic disorders (pain, swelling, tenderness in extremities, headache, chest pain, blurred vision).
- Instruct patient to notify health care professional if pregnancy is suspected.
- Caution patient to use sunscreen and protective clothing to prevent photosensitivity reactions.
- Emphasize the importance of routine follow-up, physical examination including BP, breast, abdomen, and pelvic examinations; and Pap smears.

DIAZEPAM

Classification

- **Therapeutic:** Antianxiety agents, anticonvulsants, sedative/hypnotics, skeletal muscle relaxants (centrally acting)
- **Pharmacologic:** Benzodiazepines.

Action

- Depresses the CNS, probably by potentiating GABA, an inhibitory neurotransmitter. Produces skeletal muscle relaxation by inhibiting spinal polysynaptic different pathways. Has anticonvulsant properties due to enhanced presynaptic inhibition.
- **Therapeutic effects:** Relief of anxiety, sedation, amnesia, skeletal muscle relaxation and decreased seizure activity.

Routes and Doses

Antianxiety

- **Adults:** 2–10 mg 2–4 times daily (PO)
- **Adults:** 2–10 mg, may repeat in 3–4hr as needed (IM, IV)

Precardioversion

- **IV (Adults):** 5–15 mg 5–10 minsprecardioversion

Pre-endoscopy

- **IV (Adults):** 2.5–20 mg
- **IM (Adults):** 5–10 mg 30 min pre-endoscopy

Status Epilepticus/Acute Seizure Activity

IV (Adults): 5 mg – 10 mg

Skeletal Muscle Relaxation:

- **Adults:** 2–10 mg 3–4 times daily (PO)
- **Geriatric Patients or Debilitated Patients:** 2–2.5 mg 1–2 times initially (PO)
- **Adults:** 5–10 mg; may repeat in 2–4 hr (IM, IV)
- **Geriatric Patients or Debilitated Patients:** 2–5 mg–4 hr. (IM, IV)

Indications

- **Adjunct in the management of:** Anxiety disorder, athetosis, anxiety relief prior to cardioversion (injection), stiffman syndrome, preoperative sedation (provides light anaesthesia and anterograde amnesia). Treatment of status epilepticus/uncontrolled seizures (injection). Skeletal muscle relaxant. Decreased seizure activity.
- **Unlabeled use:** Anxiety associated with acute myocardial infarction, insomnia.

Contraindications

Hypersensitivity, cross sensitivity with other benzodiazepines may occur, comatose patients, myasthenia gravis, severe pulmonary impairment, sleep apnea, severe hepatic dysfunction, pre-existing CNS depression, uncontrolled severe pain, angle-closure glaucoma, some products contain alcohol, propylene, glycol or tartrazine and should be avoided in patients with known hypersensitivity or intolerance;

- **Obstetrics:** Increased risk of congenital malformations
- **Pediatrics:** Children less than 6 months (for Oral; safety not established)
- **Lactation:** Recommended to discontinue drug or bottle- feed
- **Use cautiously in:** Severe renal impairment, History of suicide attempt or drug dependence, debilitated patients (dose reduction required) and patients with low albumin
- **Pediatric:** Metabolites can accumulate in neonates
- **GERI:** Long-acting benzodiazepines cause prolonged sedation in the elderly, appears on Beers list and is associated with increased risk of falls (Decrease dose required or consider short-acting benzodiazepine).

Side Effects

- **CNS:** Dizziness, drowsiness, lethargy, depression, hangover, ataxia, slurred speech, headache, paradoxical excitation
- **EENT:** Blurred vision
- **Respiratory:** Respiratory depression
- **CVS:** Hypotension (IV only)
- **GI:** Constipation, diarrhea (may be caused by propylene glycol content in oral solution), nausea, vomiting, weight gain
- **Dermatology:** Rashes
- **Local:** Pain (IM), phlebitis (IV), venous thrombosis
- **Miscellaneous:** Physical dependence, tolerance.

Nursing Assessment and Management

Assessment

- Monitor blood pressure, pulse, and respiratory rate prior to and periodically throughout therapy and frequently during IV therapy
- Assess IV site frequently during administration; diazepam may cause phlebitis and venous thrombosis
- Prolonged high-dose therapy may lead to psychological or physical dependence. Restrict amount of drug available to patient. Observe depressed patients closely for suicidal tendencies

- Conduct regular assessment of continued need for treatment
- **Geriatrics:** Assess risk for falls and institute fall prevention strategies
- **Anxiety:** Assess mental status (orientation, mood, behavior) and degree of anxiety
- Assess level of sedation (ataxia, dizziness, slurred speech) prior to and periodically throughout therapy
- **Seizures:** Observe and record intensity, duration and location of seizure activity. The initial dose diazepam offers seizure control for 15–20 minutes after administration. Institute seizure precautions
- **Muscle:** Assess muscle spasm, associated pain, and limitation of movement prior to and during therapy.

Management

- Instruct patient to take medication as directed and not take more than prescribed or increase dose if less effective after a few weeks without checking with health care professional.
- Medication may cause drowsiness, clumsiness or unsteadiness. Advise patient to avoid driving or other activities requiring alertness until response to medication is known
- Caution patient to avoid taking alcohol or other CNS depressants concurrently with this medication.
- Advise patient to notify health care professional, if pregnancy is planned or suspected
- Emphasize the importance of follow up examinations to determine effectiveness of the medications.

PHENYTOIN

Classification

- **Therapeutic:** Antiarrhythmics (group IB), anticonvulsant
- **Pharmacologic:** Hydantoins.

Action

- Limits seizure propagation by altering ion transport. May also decrease synaptic transmission. Antiarrhythmic properties as a results of shorting the action potential and decreasing automaticity
- **Therapeutic effect:** Diminished seizure activity. Termination of ventricular arrhythmias.

Routes and Doses

IM administration is not recommended due to erratic absorption and pain on injection.

Anticonvulsant

- **Adults:** PO, Loading does of 15–20 mg/kg as extended capsule in divided dose is given every 2–4 hrly; maintenance does 5–6 mg/kg/day given in 1–3 divided does; usual dosing range = 200–1200 mg/day
- **Children 10–16 years:** PO, 6–7 mg/kg/day in 2–3 divided dose
- **Children 7–9 years:** PO, 7–8 mg/kg/day in 2 -3 divided does
- **Children 4–6 years:** PO, 7.5–9 mg/kg/day in 2–3 divided does
- **Children 0.5–3 years:** PO, 8–10 mg/kg/day in 2–3 divided dose
- **Neonates up to 6 months:** PO, 5–8 mg/kg/day in divided dose, may require q 8 hr dosing
- **Adult:** IV, 15–20 mg/kg at 1–3 mg/kg/min. Maintenance dose - same as PO dosing above
- **Children:** IV, 15–20 mg/kg.

Antiarrhythmic

- **Adults:** IV, 50–100 mg q 10-15 min until arrhythmias is abolished or a total of 15 mg/kg has been given or toxicity occurs
- **Adult:** PO, 250 mg QID for 1 day then 250 mg BID for 2 days then maintenance at 300–400 mg/day in divided dose
- **Children:** IV, 1.25 mg/kg q 5 min may repeat dose up to 15 mg/kg. Maintenance does 5–10 mg/kg/day in 2-3 divided dose IV or PO.

Indications

- **Treatment/prevention of tonic:** Clonic (grand mal) seizure and complex partial seizure
- **Unlabeled use:** As an antiarrhythmic, particularly for ventricular arrhythmias associated with digoxin toxicity, prolonged QT interval, and surgical repair of congenital heart disease in children
- Management of neuropathic pain, including trigeminal neuralgia.

Contraindications

Hypersensitivity, hypersensitivity to propylene glycol (phenytoin injection only), alcohol intolerance (phenytoin injection and liquid only), sinus bradycardia, sinoatrial block, 2nd or 3rd degree heart block, or Stokes Adams syndrome (phenytoin injection only).

- **Use cautiously in** all patients hepatic or renal disease, patients with severe cardiac or respiratory diseases
- **Obstetric:** Safety not established; may results in fetal hydantoin syndrome if used chronically or hemorrhage in the newborn if used at term; use with extreme caution
- **Lactation:** Safety not established
- **Pediatric:** Suspension contain sodium benzoate, metabolite of benzyl alcohol that can cause potentially fetal gasping syndrome in neonates
- **Geriatric:** Use of IV phenytoin may results in an increased risk of serious adverse reaction.

Side Effects

- **CNS:** Suicidal thought, ataxia, agitation, confusion, dizziness, drowsiness, dysarthria, dyskinesia, extrapyramidal syndrome, headache, insomnia, weakness
- **EENT:** Diplopia and nystagmus
- **CV:** Hypotension and tachycardia
- **GI:** Gingival hyperplasia, nausea, constipation, drug-induced hepatitis, vomiting
- **Dermatology:** Hypertrichosis, rash, exfoliative dermatitis, pruritus, purple glove syndrome
- **Hematology:** Agranulocytosis, aplastic anemia, leukopenia, megaloblastic anemia, thrombocytopenia
- **MS:** Osteomalacia, osteoporosis
- **Miscellaneous:** Allergic reaction including Stevens -Johnson syndrome, fever lymphadenopathy.

Nursing Assessment and Management

Assessment

- Monitored closely change in behavior that could indicate the emergence or worsening of suicidal thought or behavior or depression

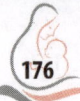

- Assess oral hygiene. Various cleaning begins within 10 days of initiation of phenytoin therapy may help control gingival hyperplasia
- Assess patients for phenytoin hypersensitivity syndrome. Rash usually occurs within the first 2 weeks of therapy
- Observed patients for development of rash. Discontinue phenytoin at the first sign of skin reaction
- **Seizure:** Assess location, duration, frequency and characteristics of seizure activity. EEG may be monitored periodically throughout therapy
- Monitored blood pressure, ECG and respiratory function continuously during administration of IV phenytoin and throughout period
- **Arrhythmias:** Monitored ECG continuously during treatment of arrhythmias
- May cause increase serum alkaline phosphatase, GGT and glucose levels
- Monitored serum folate concentrations periodically during prolonged therapy.

INDOMETHACIN

Classification

Therapeutic: Antirheumatics, ductus arteriosus patency adjuncts (IV Only), nonsteroidal anti-inflammatory agents.

Action

- Inhibits prostaglandin synthesis
- **Therapeutic effects:** Suppression of pain and inflammation (PO), Closure of PDA (IV).

Routes and Doses

- **Anti-inflammatory**
- **PO (Adult)**
- **Antiarthritic:** 25–50 mg 2–4 times daily or 75 mg once or twice daily
- **Antigout:** 100 mg initially, followed by 50 mg 3 times daily
- **PO (Children>2 yrs):** 1–2 mg/kg/day in 2 divided doses.
- **PDA Closure:**
- **IV (Neonates):** 0.2 mg/kg initially, then 2 subsequent doses at 12–24 hour interval of 0.1 mg/kg if age>48 hour at time of initial dose; 0.2 mg/kg if 2–7days at initial dose; 0.25 mg/kg if age>7 days at initial dose.

Indication

- **PO: Inflammatory disorders including:** Rheumatoid arthritis, Gouty arthritis, Osteoarthritis, Ankylosing spondylitis. Generally reserved for patients who do not respond to less toxic agents.
- **IV:** Alternative to surgery in the management of patent ductus arteriosus (PDA) in premature neonates.

Contraindication

- **Contraindicated in:** Hypersensitivity; known alcohol intolerance (suspension), cross-sensitivity may exist with other NSAIDS, including aspirin, active GI bleeding, ulcer disease, proctitis or recent history of rectal bleeding, intraventricular hemorrhage, thrombocytopenia, Pediatric Increases risk of necrotizing enterocolitis and bowel perforation in premature infants with PDA.

- **Use cautiously in** severe cardiovascular, renal or hepatic disease, History of ulcer diseases, Epilepsy, Hypertension
- **Obstetric:** Not recommended during 2nd half of pregnancy lactation, increased risk of adverse reactions.

Side Effects

- **CNS:** Dizziness, drowsiness, headache, psychic disturbances
- **EENT:** Blurred vision, tinnitus
- **CVS:** Hypertension, edema
- **GI:** Drug induced hepatitis GI bleeding, constipation, dyspepsia, colitis.
- **GU:** Cystitis, hematuria, renal failure
- **Dermatology:** Rashes; F and E: hypercalcemia, dilutional hyponatremia, hypoglycemia
- **Hematology:** Bleeding time
- **Local:** Phlebitis at IV site
- **Miscellaneous:** Allergic reactions including Anaphylaxis.

Nursing Assessment and Management

- Patients who have asthma, aspirin-induced allergy and nasal polyps are at increases risk for developing hypersensitivity reactions
- Monitor for rhinitis, asthma and urticarial
- Assess limitation of movement and pain
- Monitor respiratory status, heart rate, blood pressure, echocardiogram and heart sounds routinely throughout therapy
- Monitor intake and output. Fluids restriction is usually instituted throughout therapy.

SALBUTAMOL

Classification

- **Therapeutic:** Bronchodilators
- **Pharmacologic:** Adrenergic.

Action

Binds to beta2- adrenergic receptors in airway smooth muscle, leading to activation of adenyl cyclase and increase levels of cyclic-3', 5' adenosine monophosphate (c-AMP). Increases in cAMP activate kinases, which inhibit the phosphorylation of myosin and decrease intracellular calcium. Decreased intracellular calcium relaxes smooth muscles airway. Relaxation of airway smooth muscles with subsequent bronchodilation.

Therapeutic effect: Bronchodilation.

Route and Dose

- **PO (Adult and Children>12 years):** 2–4 mg 3–4 times a day
  - **Geriatric patients:** 2 mg 3–4 times a day
  - **Children 6 –12 years:** 2 mg 3–4 times daily
  - **Children 2–6 years:** 0.1 mg/kg 3 times daily.

- **Inhale (Adults and Children > 4 years):** 2 inhalation q 4–6 hourly
  - **Adults and Children > 12 years:** 2.5–5 mg q 20 mins for 3 doses
  - **Adults and Children 2–12 years:** 0.15 mg/kg/dose q 20 mins for 3 doses.

Indications

- Used as bronchodilator to control and prevent reversible airway obstruction caused by asthma or COPD.
- **Inhale:** Used as a quick- relief agent for acute bronchospasm
- **PO:** Used as a long-term control agent in patients with chronic/persistent bronchospasm.

Contraindication

Hypersensitivity.

Use cautiously in: Cardiac disease, hypertension, diabetes, glaucoma, seizure disorder, excess inhaler use may lead to tolerance and paradoxical bronchospasm.

Side Effects

- **CNS:** Nervousness, restlessness, tremor and headache
- **Respiratory:** Paradoxical bronchospasm
- **CV:** Chest pain and palpitations
- **GI:** Nausea and vomiting
- **Endo:** Hypertension
- **F and E:** Hyperkalemia
- **Neurology:** Tremor.

Nursing Assessment and Management

- Assess for lung sounds, pulse and blood pressure before administration
- Assess for amount, color and character of sputum
- Monitor pulmonary function test before initiating therapy and periodically during therapy
- Observe for paradoxical bronchospasm (wheezing).

TERBUTALINE

Classification

- **Therapeutic:** Bronchodilators and tocolytic
- **Pharmacologic:** Adrenergics.

Action

Results in the accumulation of cyclic adenosine monophosphate (CAMP) at beta –adrenergic receptors. Produces bronchodilation. Inhibits the release of mediators of immediate hypersensitivity reactions from mast cell. Relatively selective for beta2-adrenergic reception sites, with less effect on beta1, - adrenergic receptors.

Therapeutic effects: Brochodilation.

Routes and Doses

- **PO (Adults and children>15 years):**
  - Bronchodilation-2.5 – 5 mg 3 times daily, given q 6 hr
  - Tocolysis 2.5 – 10 mg q 4–6 hr until delivery (unlabelled).
- **Children 12–15 years:** PO, Bronchodialtion 2.5 mg 3 times daily (given q 6 h)
- **Children <12 years:** PO, Bronchodilation 0.05 mg/kg 3 times daily
- **Subcutaneous (Adult and children >12 years):** Bronchodilation – 250 mg
- **Subcutaneous (children ≥ 12 years):** Bronchodilation 0.005 – 0.01 mg/kg.
- **Adults:** IV, Tocolysis- 2.5 – 10 mcg/min infusion. ↑ by 5 mcg/min q 10 min until contractions stop. After contractions have stopped for 30 min ↓ infusion rate to lowest effective amount and maintain for 4–8 hours.

Availability

- **Tablets:** 2.5 mg, 5 mg
- **Injection:** 1 mg/ml.

Indications

Management of reversible airway disease due to asthma or COPD; inhalation and subcut used for short-term control and oral agent as long–term control.

Unlabeled use: Management of pre-term labor (tocolytic).

Contraindications

- Hypersensitivity to adrenergic amines.
- **Use Cautiously in:** Cardiac disease, hypertension, hyperthyroidism, diabetes, glaucoma
- **Geriatric:** More susceptible to adverse reactions, may require dose ↓ excessive use may lead to tolerance and par); adoxical bronchospasm (inhaler OB, Lactation: Pregnancy (near term) and lactation.

Side Effects

- **CNS:** Restlessness, tremor, headache, insomnia and Nervousness
- **CV:** Angina, arrhythmias, hypertension and tachycardia.
- **GI:** Nausea vomiting,
- **Endocrine:** Hyperglycemia

Nursing Assessment and Management

Assessment

- **Bronchodilator:**
  - Assess lung sounds, respiratory pattern, pulse and blood pressure before administration and during peak of medication
  - Note amount, color and character of sputum produced and notify health care professionals of abnormal findings

- Monitor pulmonary function tests before initiating therapy and periodically throughout therapy to determine effectiveness of medication.
- **Preterm Labor:**
  - Monitor maternal pulse and blood pressure, frequency and duration of contractions and fetal heart rate
  - Notify health care professional if contractions persists or increase in frequency or duration or if symptoms of maternal or fetal distress occur
  - Maternal side effects include tachycardia, palpitations, tremor, anxiety and headache
  - Assess maternal respiratory status for symptoms of pulmonary edema
  - Monitor mother and neonate for symptoms of hypoglycemia and mother for hypokalemia
  - Monitor maternal serum glucose and electrolytes.

LAMIVIUDINE

Classification

- **Therapeutic:** Antiretrovirals, antivirals
- **Pharmacologic:** Nucleoside reverse transcriptase inhibitor.

Action

After intracellular conversion to its active form, inhibits viral DNA synthesis by inhibiting the enzyme reverse transcriptase

Therapeutic effects: Slows the progression of HIV infection and decreases the occurrence of its sequelae. Increases CD4 cell counts and decreases viral load. Protection from liver damage caused by chronic hepatitis B infection; decreases viral load.

Routes and Doses

- **Route:** Oral
- **Dose and frequency:** Oral 150 mg twice daily or 300 mg once daily
- **Indication:** HIV infection. Chronic hepatitis B infection
- **Contraindication:** Hypersensitivity
- **Lactation:** Breastfeeding not recommended for HIV positive mothers.

Side Effects

- **CNS:** Seizure, fatigue, headache, insomnia, malaise, depression and dizziness
- **Resp:** Cough
- **GI:** Anorexia, diarrhea, nausea, vomiting, abdominal discomfort, abnormal liver function studies and dyspepsia
- **Dermatology:** Alopecia, rashes and urticaria
- **Endocrinology:** Hyperglycemia
- **Hematology:** Anemia, neutropenia, pure red cell aplasia
- **MS:** Musculoskeletal pain, muscle weakness.
- **Neurology:** Neuropathy.
- **Miscellaneous:** Hypersensitivity.

Nursing Assessment and Management

Assessment

- **HIV:** Assess patient for changes in severity of symptoms of HIV infection and for symptoms of opportunistic infection during therapy
- Monitor patient for sign and symptoms of periphereal neuropathy
- Assess patients for signs of pancreatitis periodically during therapy. May required discontinuation of therapy
- Monitor sings of hepatitis during therapy
- Monitor liver function test
- May rarely cause neutropenia and anemia
- Monitor serum amylase, lipase, and triglycerides periodically during therapy. Elevated level may indicate pancreatitis and require discontinuation.

Nursing Diagnosis

- Risk for infection.

Implementation

- Do not confuse lamivudine with lamotrigine. Do not confuse Epivir tablets and oral solution with Epivir-HIV tablets
- Orally may be administered without regard to food.

Patient/Family Teaching

- Instruct patient to take medicine as directed every 12 hour. Explain the difference between Epivir and Epivir-HIV to patient
- Take missed doses as soon as possible unless almost time for the next dose. Do not double dose. Caution patient not to share medication with others
- Inform patient that lamivudine does not cure HIV disease. It does not reduce risk of transmission of HIV to others through sexual contact or blood contamination. Caution patient to use condom during sexual contact and avoid sharing needle
- Instruct patient to notify health care professional promptly if signs of peripheral neuropathy or pancreatitis occur
- Advice patient not to take other treatment like herbal products without consulting health care professional
- Emphasize the importance of regular follow-up exams and blood tests to determine progress and monitor for side effects.

NONETHISTERONE

Classification

Therapeutic: Contraceptive hormones.

Action

Provide a fixed dosage of estrogen over 21 days of cycle, inhibit ovulation; may also alter tubal transport of sperm egg and prevent implant.

Therapeutic effects: Prevention of pregnancy. Decreased severity of acne. Decrease in menstrual blood loss. Decrease in premenstrual disphoric disorder.

Routes and Doses

- **Route:** Oral
- **Dose and frequency:** On 21 day regimen, take first tablet on first day after menses begins for 21 days, then skip 7 days and begin again
- **Indication:** Prevention of pregnancy. Regulation of menstrual cycle. Emergency contraception. Treatment of heavy menstrual bleeding in women who choose to use intrauterine contraception as method of contraception. Treatment of premenstrual dysphoric disorder. Management of acne in women.

Contraindication

- **Obstetric:** Pregnancy, history of thromboembolic disease, valvular heart disease, uncontrolled hypertension, multiple sexual partners, abnormal genital bleeding and liver disease
- **Lactation:** Avoid use.

Side Effects

- **CNS:** Headache and depression
- **CV:** Hypertension, edema and thromboembolic phenomena
- **GI:** Nausea, vomiting, abdominal cramps, bloating, jaundice and gallbladder disease
- **GU:** Amenorrhea, breakthrough bleeding, dysmenorrheal and spotting
- **Dermatology:** Rashes and melasma
- **Endocrinology:** Hyperglycemia
- **MS:** Musculoskeletal pain and muscle weakness
- **Miscellaneous:** Hypersensitivity, weight loss.

NURSING ASSESSMENT AND MANAGEMENT

Assessment

- Assess blood pressure before and periodically during therapy
- **ACNE:** Asses skin lesion before and after periodically during therapy
- Monitor hepatic function periodically during therapy.

Nursing Diagnosis

Non compliance.

Implementation

- Oral doses may be administered with or immediately after food to reduce nausea. Chewable tablets may be swallowed whole or chewed; if chewed follow 8 ounces of liquid
- **Subcut:** Shake vigorously before use to form a uniform suspension. Inject slowly at 45° angle into fatty area, do not rub
- **Intrauterine system:** Should be inserted by a trained heath care provider.

Patient Family Teaching

- Instruct patient to take oral medication as directed at the same time each day. Pills should be taken in proper sequence and kept in the original container. Advice patient not to skip pills even if not having sex very often

- Advise patient taking extended cycle tablets that spotting or bleeding may occur, especially after 3 months
- Advise patient of the need to use another form of Contraception for the first 3 week when beginning to use oral contraceptives
  - Advice patient that a second method of birth control should also be used during each cycle
  - Explain dose schedule and maintenance routine. Discontinuing medicine suddenly may cause withdrawal bleeding
- If nausea becomes a problem advise patient that eating solid food often provides relief
- Advise patient to report signs of fluid retention, tenderness in extremities, headache, mental depression, hepatic dysfunction
- Instruct patient to stop medicine, if pregnancy is suspected.

TETANUS TOXOID

Classification

- **Pharmacologic classification:** Toxoid
- **Therapeutic classification:** Tetanus prophylaxis
- *Pregnancy risk category C*

Indication

- Primary immunization for children under 7 yrs of age consist of 5 doses of vaccine
- It is indicated for booster injection and older against tetanus.

Routes and Dosages

- **Adult:** IM/SC- Primary immunization: 3 doses (0.5 mL each of tetanus toxoid adsorbed) via IM administration
- Give 2nd dose 4–8 weeks after 1st dose and 3rd dose 6–12 month after 2nd dose, Booster dose: 0.5 mL.

Contraindications and precautions

- Contraindicated in immunosuppressed patients and in those with immunoglobulin abnormalities or severe hypersensitivity or neurologic reactions to the toxoid or its ingredients (such as thimerosal)
- Also contraindicated in patients with thrombocytopenia or any coagulation disorder that would contraindicate IM injection unless the potential benefits outweigh the risks.

Use cautiously in:

- Cerebral damage, Neurologic disorder, History of febrile seizure
- History of Guillain-Barre syndrome
- Immune system disorder
- Illness/Infection
- High fever previous vaccination.

Adverse reactions/Side effects

- **CNS:** Headache, *seizures,* malaise, slight fever, aches and pains
- **CV:** *Tachycardia, hypotension,* flushing

- **Skin:** Urticaria, pruritus, erythema, induration and nodule (at injection site)
- **Other:** Chills, *anaphylaxis.*

Nursing Assessment and Management

- Adsorbed toxoids induce higher antitoxin titers and more persistent antitoxin levels
  - **Alert** Monitor patient for hypersensitivity reactions, seizures, and injection site reactions
  - **Alert have epinephrine** 1: 1, 000 solution available to treat allergic reactions
- Don't confuse drug with tetanus immune globulin
- Refrigerate at 36° to 46° F (2° to 8° C). Don't freeze.

Pregnant patients

- Although there is no evidence of teratogenicity, it is recommended that administration be deferred until second trimester.

Breastfeeding patients

- It is not known whether tetanus toxoid appears in breast milk. Use cautiously in breastfeeding women.

Pediatric patients

- Tetanus toxoid and tetanus toxoid adsorbed are not indicated for children younger than age 7. The vaccine is suitable for children ages 6 weeks to 6 years; however,

Geriatric patients

- These patients develop lower antitoxin levels than younger patients after tetanus immunization; therefore, skin test responsiveness may be delayed or reduced.

Patient education

- Inform patient of possible adverse reactions
- Encourage patient to report distressing adverse reactions
- Tell patient that immunization requires a series of injections. Stress the importance of keeping scheduled appointments for subsequent doses.
- Reactions may be *common*, uncommon, *life-threatening*, or **common and life threatening**.

CERVIPRIME (DINOPROSTONE)

Classification

Therapeutic: Hormones
Pharmacologic: Prostaglandins

Action

PGE_2 promotes myometrial contractility and PGE_2 induces labor with cervical effacement and dilatation. It promotes myometrial contraction.

Therapeutic effects

It acts on predominantly on the myometrium while PGE_2 acts mainly on the cervix due to its collagenolytic property.

Routes and Doses

Gel: 0.5 mg into cervical canal or 1–2 mg in the posterior fornix.

Indications

Use in obstetrics
- Induction of labor
- Termination of molar pregnancy
- Induction of labor
- Cervical ripening prior to induction of labor,

Contraindications

- Hypersentivity
- Uterine scar, active cardiac pulmonary and renal hepatic disease.
- Hypotension and bronchial asthma

Side Effects

- Hyper stimulation of uterus. Fetal heart rate changes and meconium passage are high
- Rupture of uterus

Nursing Assessment and Management

- Assess for history and physical examination
- Monitor fetal heart sound and uterine contraction
- Monitor cervical dilation
- Monitor Bishop's scale
- Ask mother to be retain same position for minimum 30 minutes after administration
- Can repeat maximum up to 3 times if induction fails.

FERROUS SULFATE

Classification

Therapeutic: Enzymatic mineral
Pharmacologic: Iron preparation

Action

Ferrous sulfate is an essential component in the formation of hemoglobin, myoglobin and enzymes. It is necessary for effective erythropoiesis and transport or utilization of oxygen.

Therapeutic effects

Increase the Hb level in the blood and prevent antepartum hemorrhage.

Routes and Doses

Dose: 2–3 mg/kg
Frequency: Once a day Route : PO

Indications

- The prevention or treatment of iron deficiency anemia due to inadequate diet,
- Pregnancy
- Blood loss.

Contraindications

Patients receiving repeated blood transfusions; anemia not due to iron deficiency

Side Effects

- Large doses may aggravate peptic ulcer, regional enteritis and ulcerative colitis.
- Severe iron poisoning
- Vomiting, severe abdominal pain, diarrhea dehydration
- Hyperventilation, pallor or cyanosis, cardiovascular collapse

Nursing Assessment and Management

- Store all forms at room temperature.
- Give between meals (empty stomach) with water but may give with meals if gastrointestinal discomfort occurs.
- Transient staining of mucous membranes and teeth will occur with liquid iron preparation.
- To avoid, place liquid on the back of the tongue with dropper or use straw.
- Avoid simultaneous administration of antacids or tetracycline.
- Do not crush sustained-release preparations.
- Eggs and milk inhibit absorption.
- Introduce vitamin C supplement to improve iron absorption eg: lime, Amla etc
- Introduce dietary supplementation of iron like jaggery, spinach, coriander leaves, dates etc
- Monitor serum iron, total iron-binding capacity, reticulocyte count, hemoglobin, and ferritin.
- Monitor daily pattern of bowel activity and stool consistency.
- Assess for clinical improvement, record of relief of symptoms (fatigue, irritability, pallor, paresthesia, and headache).

BETAMETHASONE

Classification

Corticosteroid

Action

Betamethasone is a corticosteroid with mainly glucocorticoid activity. It prevents and controls inflammation by controlling the rate of protein synthesis, depressing the migration of poly-morphonuclear leukocytes and fibroblasts, and reversing capillary permeability and lysosomal stabilization

Therapeutic Effects

It helps in the lung maturity of fetus inside the womb.

Routes and Doses

12 mg IM maximum of 2 doses.

Indications

Anticipating preterm delivery

Contraindication

Hypersensitivity; systemic fungal or acute infections

Side Effects

Hypokalemia, depression insomnia hirsutism, heart failure, fluid retention, diabetes mellitus, nausea, vomiting, pancreatitis, hypotension and acne.

Nursing Assessment and Management

- Assess for the preterm delivery
- Assess for history and physical examination
- Monitor dosages and fetal wellbeing
- Monitor for signs and symptoms of labor
- Do not administer during breastfeeding.

DUVADILAN

Classification

Vasodilator, Smooth muscle relaxant.

Brand Name: Duvadilan
Pharmacological name: Isoxsuprine

Action

Chemically similar to sympathomimetic amines and often described as beta adrenergic agonist. However, the drug appears to be a muscular tropic vasodilator and its effects are not blocked by propanolol.

Therapeutic effects

Inhibits uterine contraction and prevent preterm labor/delivery

Dose and Route

10 mg, IM

Indication

Peripheral and cerebral vascular insufficiency with spastic component showing symptoms:

- Dizziness
- Forgetfulness
- Confusion

- Visual, auditory and speech abnormalities
- Coldness and numbness of limbs
- Color changes and ischemic ulcers
- Uterine hypermotility disorders
- Threatened abortion
- Premature labor
- Dysmenorrheal

Contraindication

Recent arterial hemorrhage, heart disease and severe anemia

- Should not be administered immediately postpartum and premature labor. Avoid parenteral administration to patients with hypotension, tachycardia, premature detachment of placenta or immediate postpartum.
- Action chemically similar to sympathomimetic amines and often described as beta adrenergic agonist. However, the drug appears to be a muscular tropic vasodilator and its effects are not blocked by propanolol.

Side Effects

Transient flushing

- Hypotension
- Rashes
- Gastrointestinal (GI) disturbances
- Maternal pulmonary edema
- Fetal tachycardia
- Transient palpitations
- Dizziness.

Nursing Assessment and Management

- Assess patient's condition before therapy. Assess potential benefits from drug therapy.
- Monitor for possible drug-induced adverse reactions:
  - Hypotension
  - Tachycardia
  - Nausea
  - Vomiting
  - Dizziness
  - Severe rash
- Inform the patient about possible side effects, adverse symptoms to report.

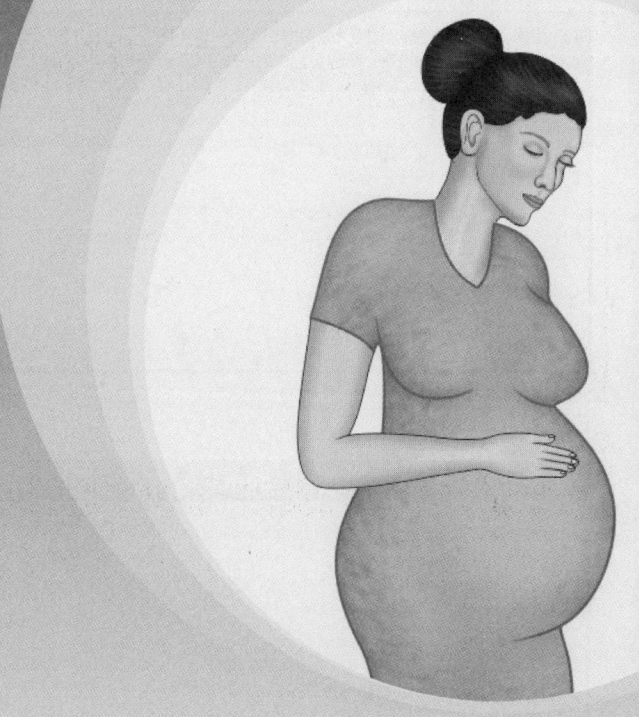

ANNEXURE

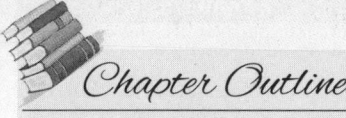

Chapter Outline

Bishop Score to Assess Cervical Favorability

Cervix	Score				Bishop Score Modifiers
	0	1	2	3	
Position	Posterior	Mid-position	Anterior		**Add 1 point for:** • Pre-eclampsia • Each previous vaginal delivery **Subtract 1 point for:** • Postdate pregnancy • Nulliparity (no previous vaginal deliveries) • PPROM (premature preterm rupture of membranes)
Consistency	Firm	Medium	Solt		
Effacement	0–30%	30–50%	60–70%	>80%	
Dilation	Closed	1–2 cm	3–4 cm	>5 cm	
Station	–3	–2	–1	+1, +2	

REEDA Scale

Points	Redness	Edema	Ecchymosis	Discharge	Approximation
0	None	None	None	None	Closed
1	Within .25 cm of incision bilaterally	Perineal, less than 1 cm, from incision	Within .25 cm bilaterally or .5 cm unilaterally	Serum	Skin separation 3 mm. or less
2	Within .5 cm of incision bilaterally	Perineal and/or Vulvar, between 1 to 2 cm, from incision	Between .25 to 1 cm bilaterally or between .5 to 2 cm unilaterally	Serosanguinous	Skin and subcutaneous fat separation
3	Beyond .5 cm of incision bilaterally	Perineal and/or Vulvar, greater than 2 cm from incision	Greater than 1 cm. bilaterally or 2 cm unilaterally	Bloody, purulent	Skin, subcutaneous fat and fascial layers separation
Score					
Total					

APGAR Scoring System

	Indicator	0 Points	1 Point	2 Points
A	Activity (muscle tone)	Absent	Flexed arms and legs	Active
P	Pulse	Absent	Below 100 bpm	Over 100 bpm
G	Grimace (reflex irritability)	Floppy	Minimal response to stimulation	Prompt response to stimulation
A	Appearance (skin color)	Blue; pale	Pink body, Blue extremities	Pink
R	Respiration	Absent	Slow and irregular	Vigorous cry

LATCH Score

	0	1	2
L Latch	Too sleepy or reluctant No latch achieved	Repeated attempts Hold nipple in mouth Stimulate to suck	Graspe breast Tongue down Lips flanged Rhythmic sucking
A Audible swallowing	None	A few with stimulation	Spontaneous and intermittent >24 hours old Spontaneous and frequent <24 hours old
T Type of nipple	Inverted	Flat	Everted (after stimulation)
C Comfort (breast/nipple)	Engorged Cracked, bleeding, large blisters or bruises Severe discomfort	Filling Reddened/small blisters or bruises Mild/moderate discomfort	Soft Nontender
H Hold (positioning)	Full assist (staff holds infant at breast)	Minimal assist (e.g., elevate head of bed, place pillows for support) Teach one side; mother does other Staff holds and than mother takes over	No assist from staff Mother able to position and hold infant

NOTE

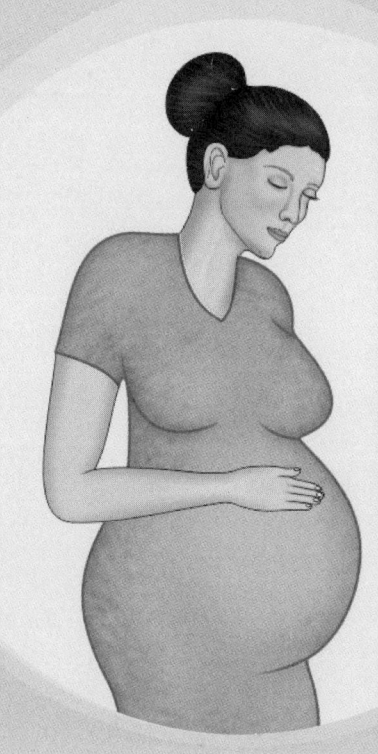

PRACTICE PARTOGHRAPH

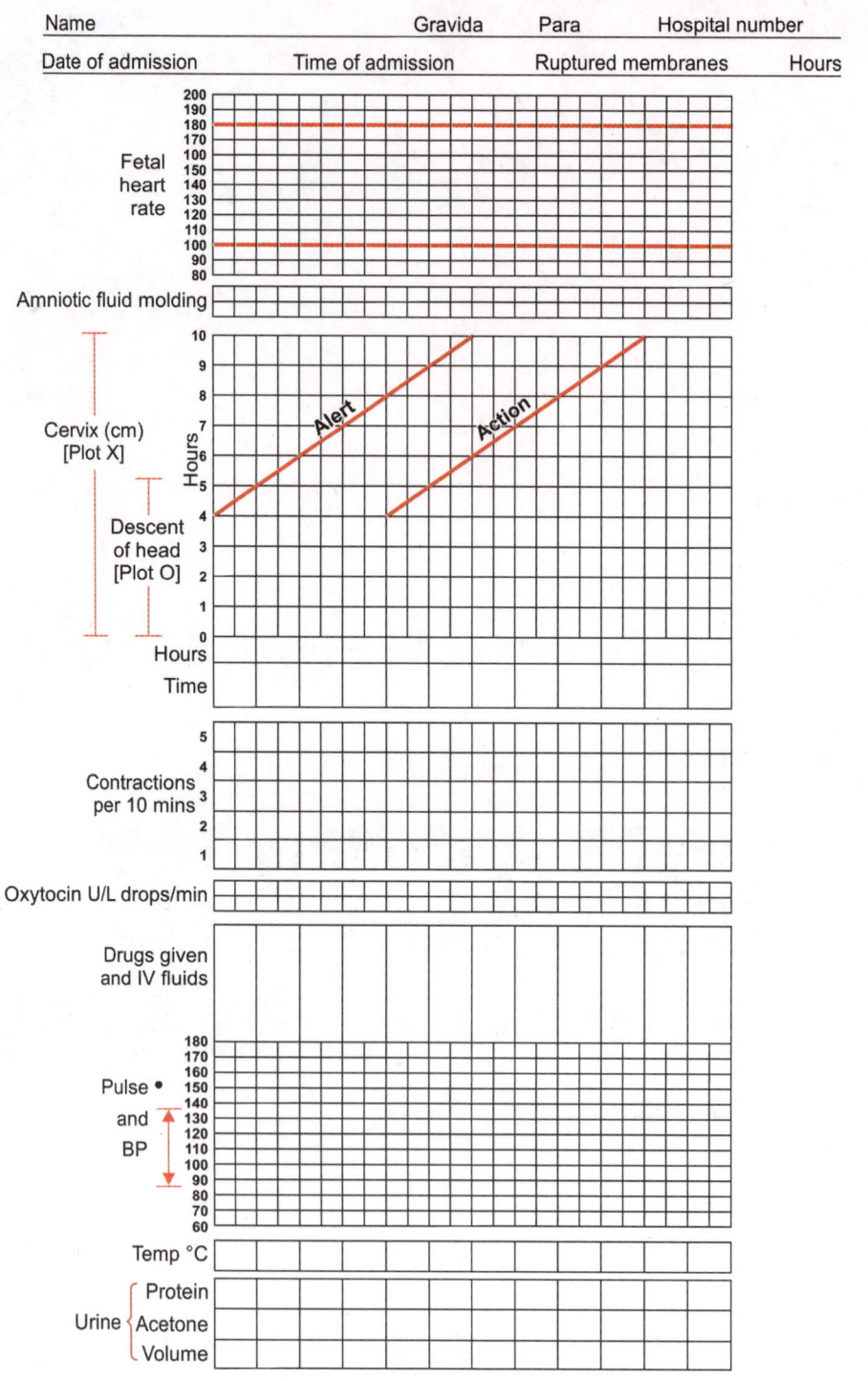

Name   Gravida   Para   Hospital number

Date of admission   Time of admission   Ruptured membranes   Hours

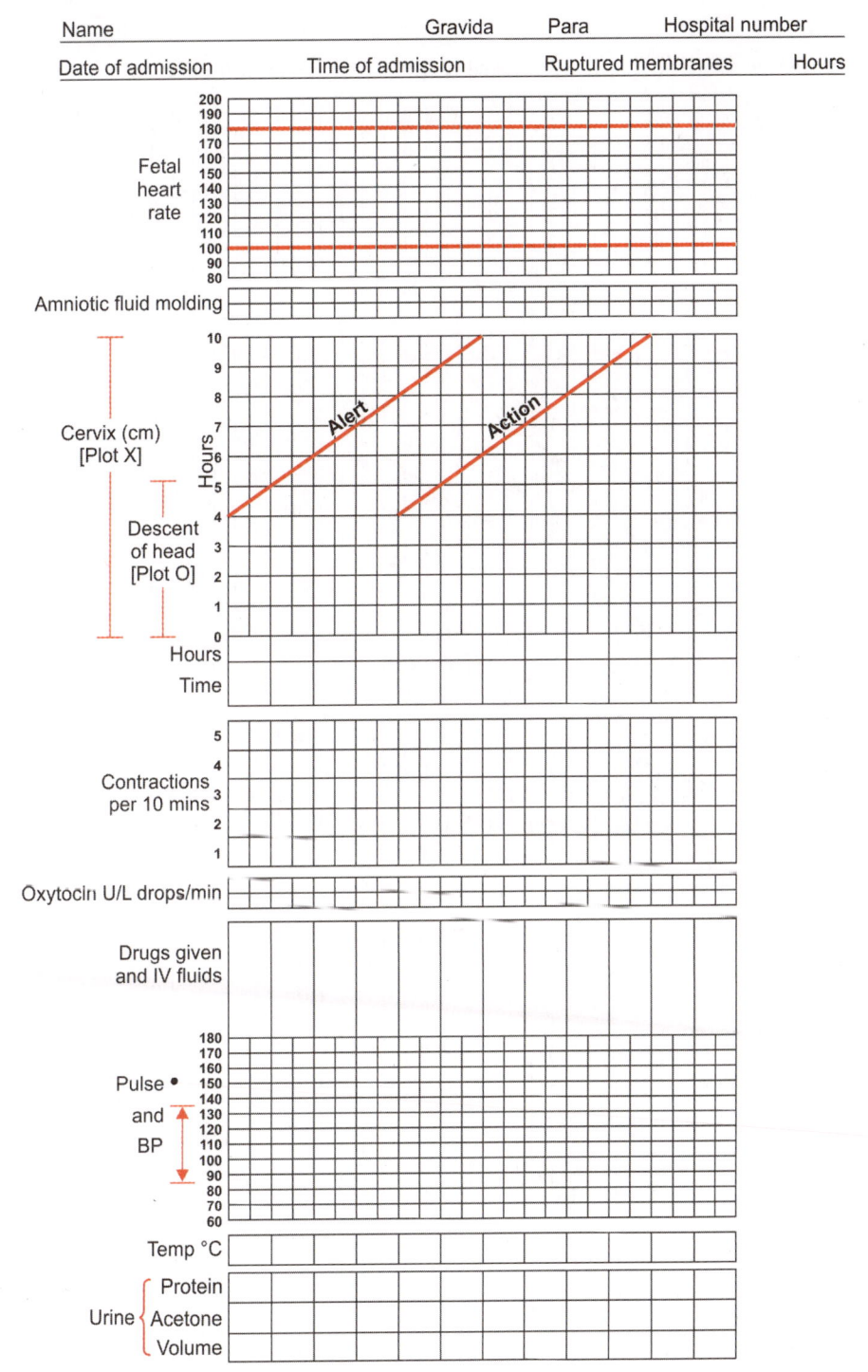

Name _____ Gravida ___ Para ___ Hospital number ___

Date of admission _____ Time of admission _____ Ruptured membranes ___ Hours ___

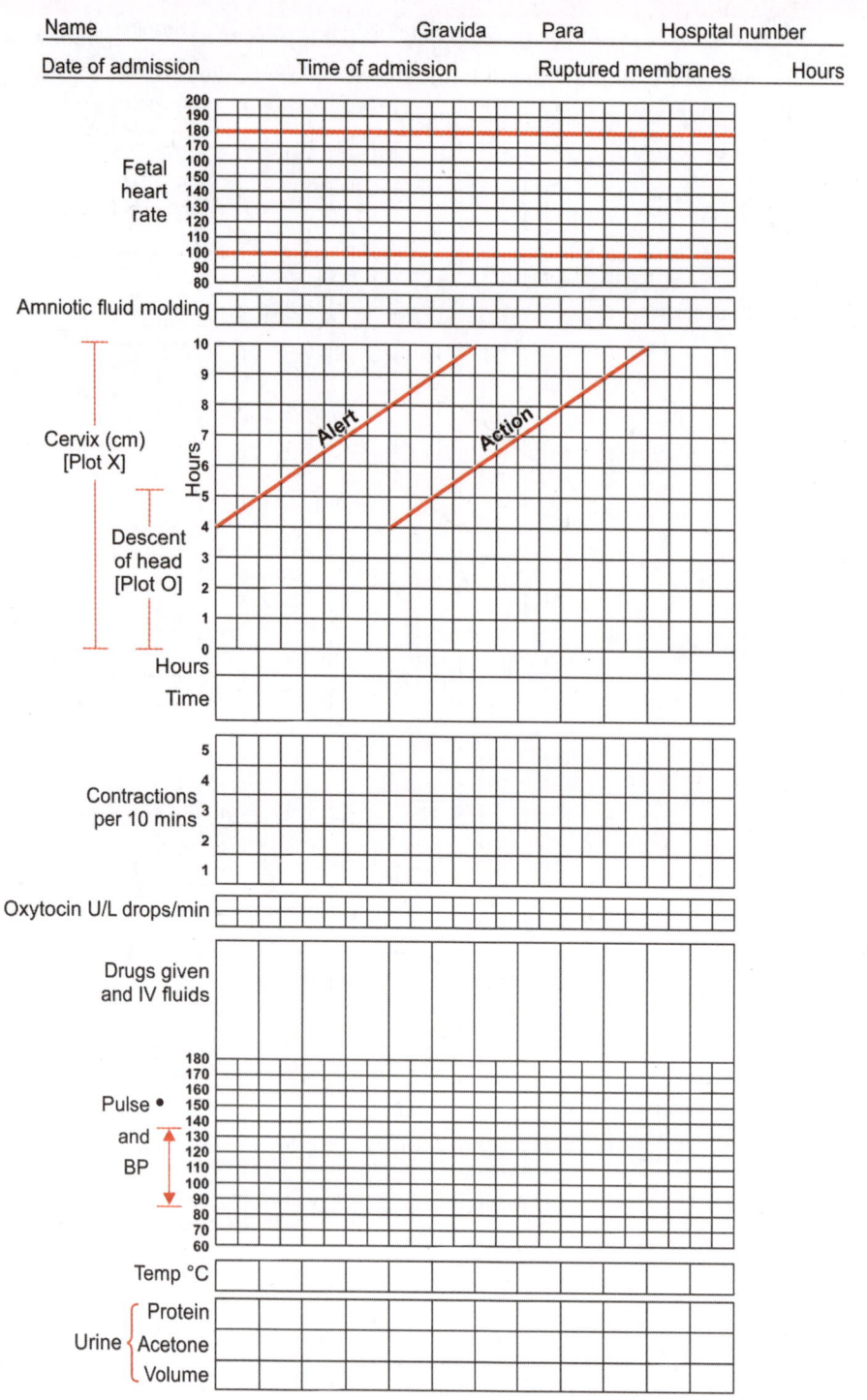

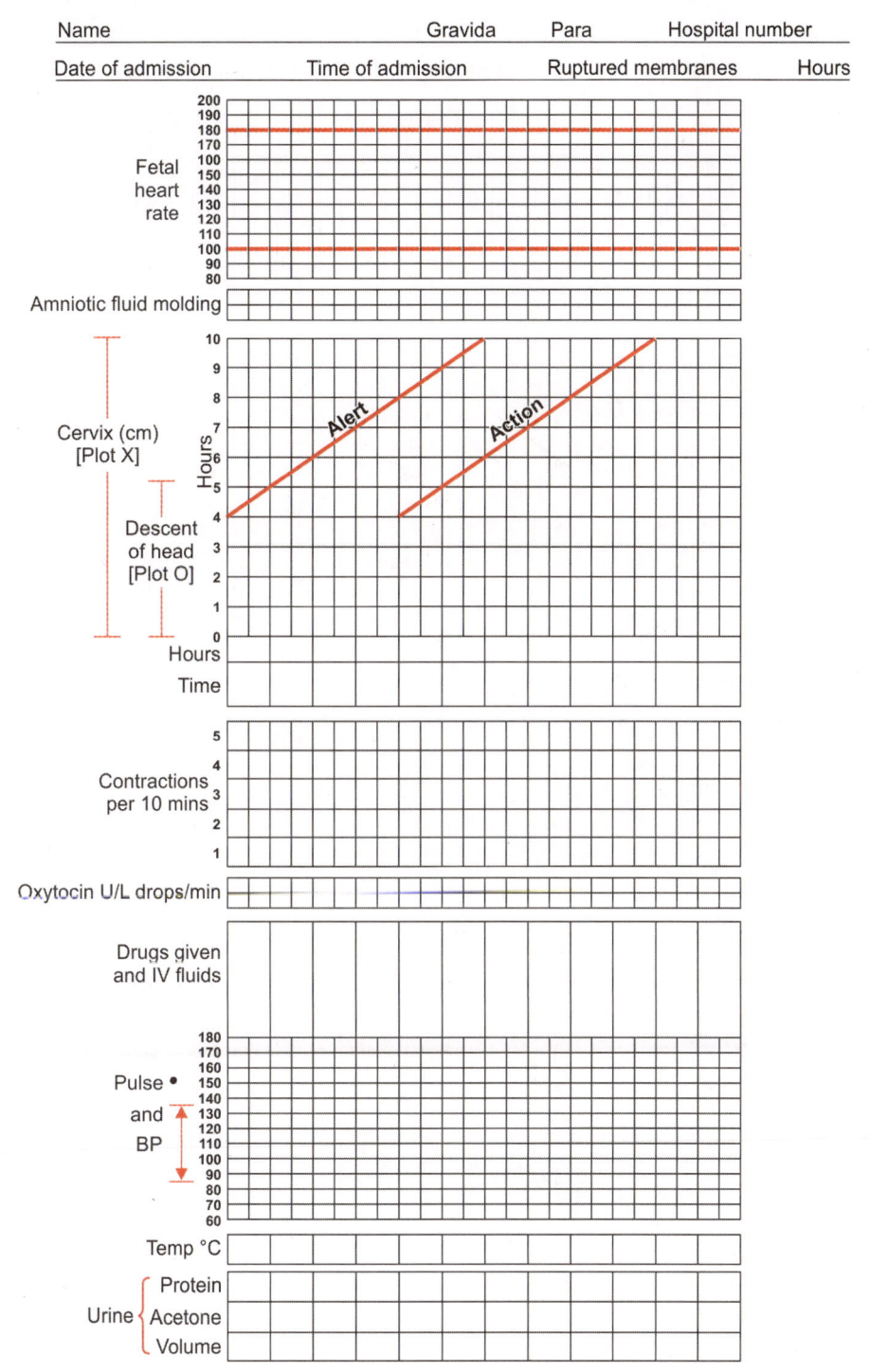

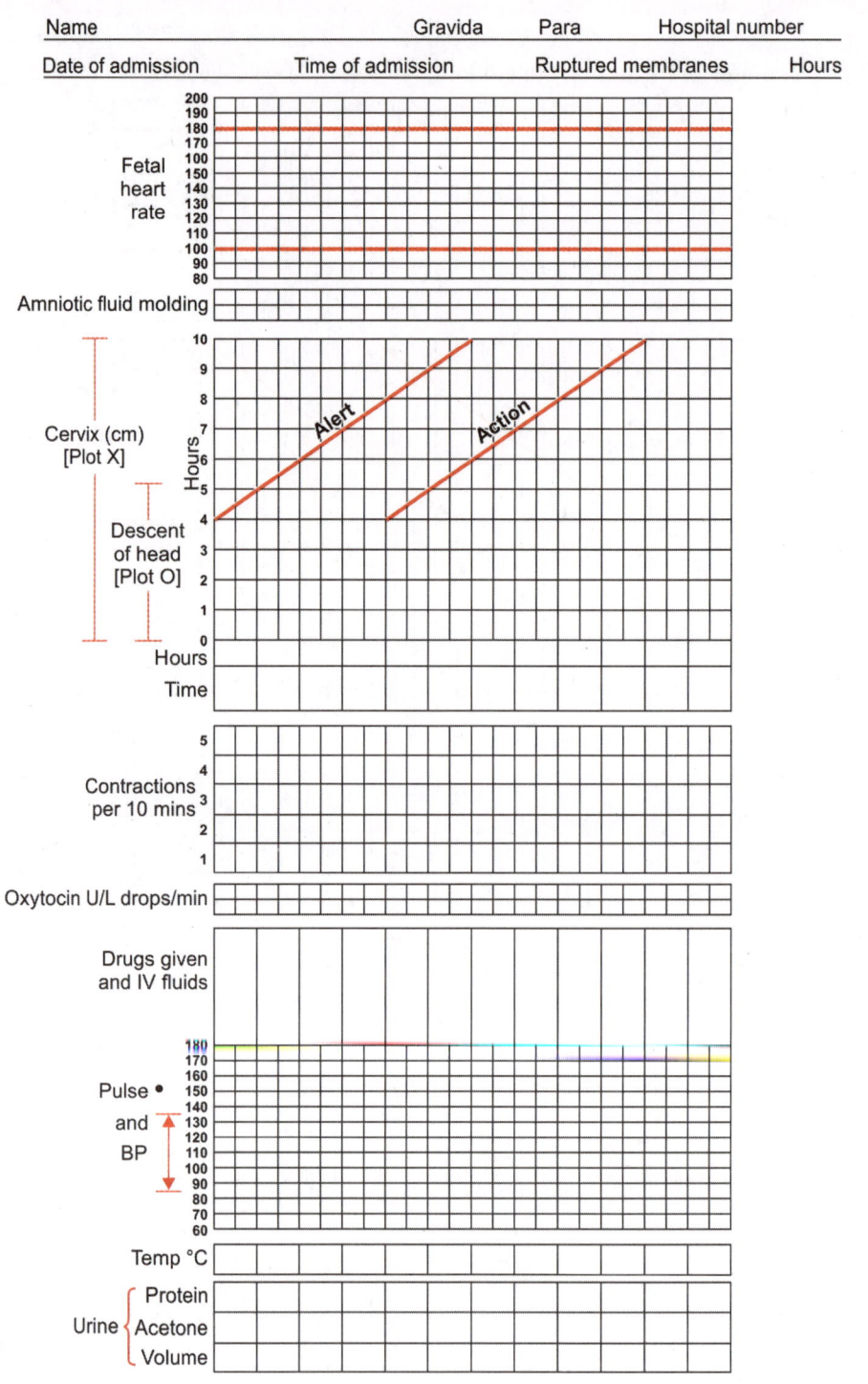

BIBLIOGRAPHY

1. Auxilliary Nurse Midwiwes Lady health Visitors and staff nurses 2010

2. Datta DC, Textbook of Obstetrics, 8th edition, New Central book agency.

3. Debdas AK. Obstetrics and Gynaecology Drug Handbook Combo, 3rd edition. New Delhi; Jaypee Brothers Publishers and Distributors. 2015

4. Devdas AK. Practical Obstetrics, 1st edition. New Delhi; Jaypee Brothers Publishers and Distributors. 2003.

5. Jacob A. Clinical Nursing Procedures: The art of Nursing Practice, 3rd edition. New Delhi; Jaypee Brothers Publishers and Distributors. 2015.

6. Jacob A. Manual of Midwifery and Gynaecological Nursing, 2nd edition. New delhi; Jaypee Brothers Publishers and Distributors Pvt Ltd.

7. Milk DL. Maternity nursing, 2nd edition. Mosby Publisher.

8. Reynolds M. Gynaecological Nursing, ELBS publisher.

9. Sandhya G, Clinical Nursing Procedures, 1st edition. New Delhi, CBS Publishers & Distributors Pvt Ltd. 2018. P. 1130.

10. Shivani S. Clinical Record Book for Midwifery, 1st edition. P V publication.

11. Turrentine JE. Clinical Protocols in Obstertics and Gynecology, volume 1, 3rd edition. London; Francis & Taylor: P. 448.

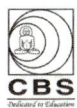

CBS

Dedicated to Education

CBS PGMEE & Nursing Division

(A Unit of CBS Publishers & Distributors Pvt. Ltd.)

Nursing Catalogue 2020

Nursing Competitive Exams, Nursing Textbooks, Record Books

Update: November, 2020

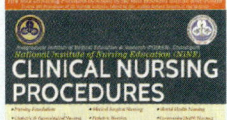
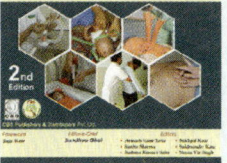

ISBN: 978-93-89261-97-4
Pages: 1296   2/e, 2019

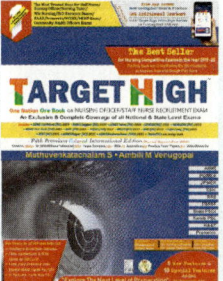

ISBN: 978-93-89261-98-1
Pages: 1350   5/e, 2020-21

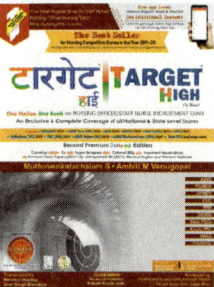

ISBN: 978-81-94025-65-8
Pages: 1296   2/e, 2020

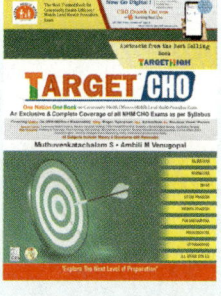

ISBN: 978-81-940256-0-3
Pages: 470   1/e, 2020

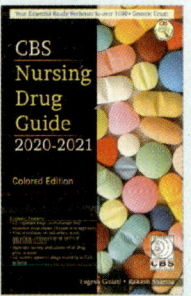

ISBN: 978-93-88178-53-2
Pages: 1670   1/e, 2020

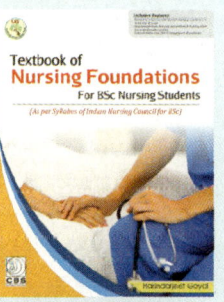

ISBN: 978-93-88108-94-2
Pages: 700   1/e, 2020

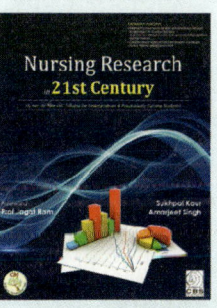

ISBN: 978-93-89261-89-9
Pages: 700   1/e, 2020

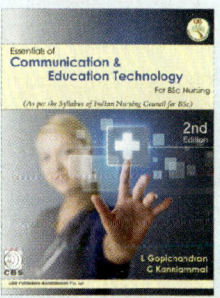

ISBN: 978-93-88178-58-7
Pages: 325   2/e, 2019

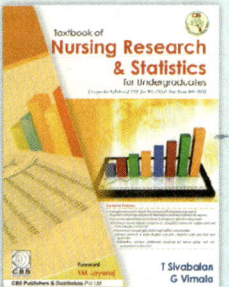

ISBN: 978-93-88178-61-7
Pages: 290   1/e, 2018

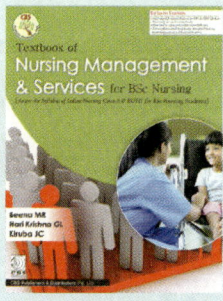

ISBN: 978-93-88178-62-4
Pages: 240   1/e, 2019

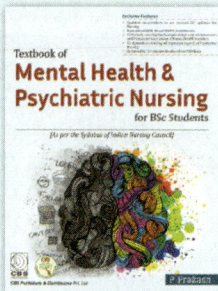

ISBN: 978-93-89261-91-2
Pages: 500   1/e, 2019

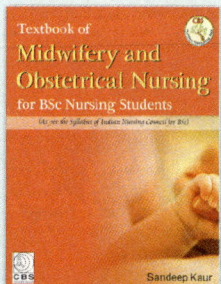

ISBN: 978-93-89261-90-5
Pages: 700 (T)   1/e, 2020

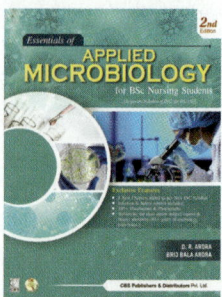

ISBN: 978-81-945234-4-4
Pages: 360   2/e, 2020-21

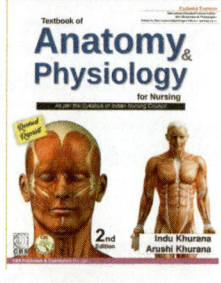

ISBN: 978-93-86827-12-8
Pages: 568   2/e, 2018

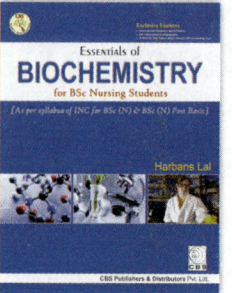

ISBN: 978-81-23927-19-0
Pages: 332   1/e (R/R), 2020-21

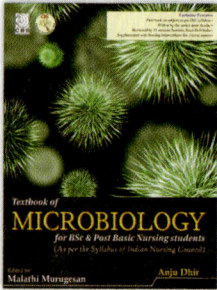

ISBN: 978-93-88108-82-9
Pages: 535   1/e, 2019

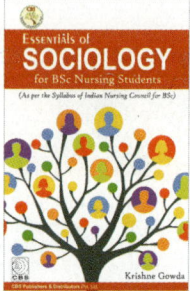

ISBN: 978-93-86217-51-6
Pages: 362   1/e, 2017

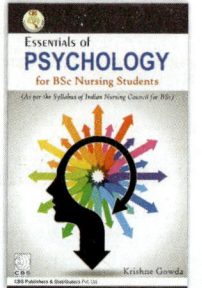

ISBN: 978-81-23927-11-4
Pages: 362   1/e, 2017-18

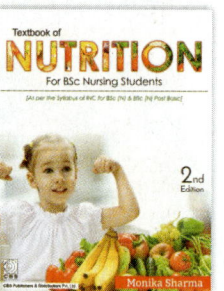

ISBN: 978-93-89261-92-9
Pages: 330   2/e, 2019

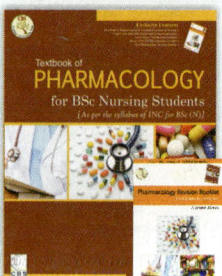

ISBN: 978-93-89261-95-0
Pages: 460   2/e, 2019

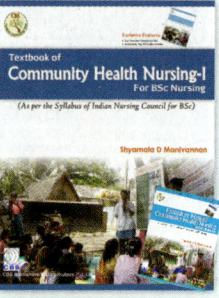

ISBN: 978-93-86217-80-6
Pages: 486   1/e, 2017-18

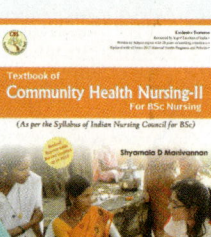
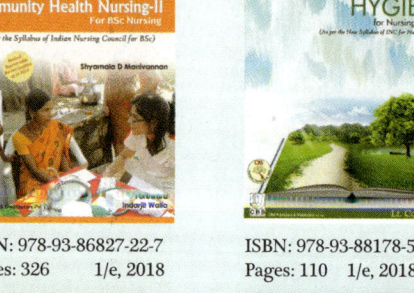

ISBN: 978-81-23927-01-5
Pages: 508   1/e, 2018

ISBN: 978-93-86827-22-7
Pages: 326   1/e, 2018

ISBN: 978-93-88178-56-3
Pages: 110   1/e, 2018-19

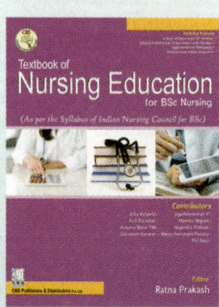

ISBN: 978-93-86827-34-0
Pages: 340   1/e, 2018

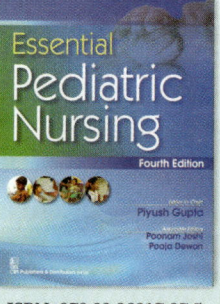

ISBN: 978-93-86217-87-5
Pages: 576   4/e, 2017

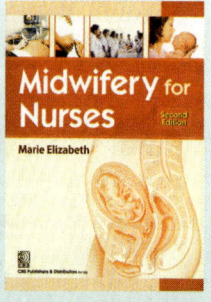

ISBN: 978-81-23922-14-0
Pages: 544   2/e, 2018

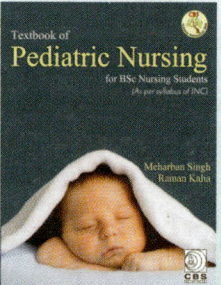

ISBN: 978-93-88108-72-0
Pages: 630   1/e, 2018

 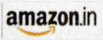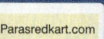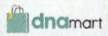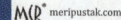

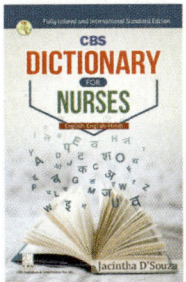

Releasing Soon

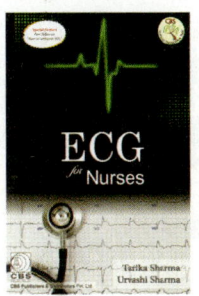

ISBN: 978-93-89261-88-2
Pages: 190   1/e, 2019

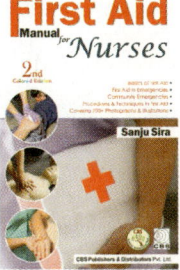

ISBN: 978-93-88178-55-6
Pages: 212   2/e, 2019

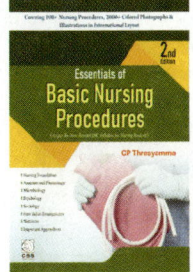

ISBN: 978-81-94523-47-5
Pages: 1016   2/e, 2020

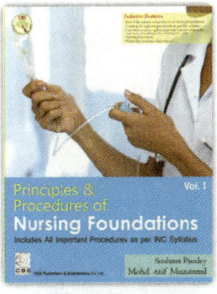

ISBN: 978-93-88108-95-9
Pages: 392   1/e, 2018

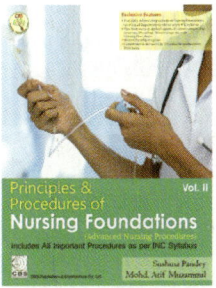

ISBN: 978-93-89261-87-5
Pages: 272   1/e, 2019

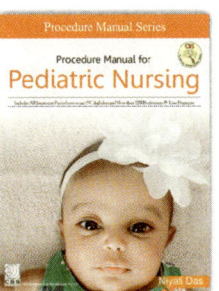

ISBN: 978-93-88108-86-7
Pages: 235   1/e, 2018

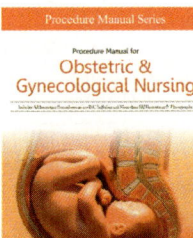

ISBN: 978-93-88178-60-0
Pages: 200   1/e, 2018-19

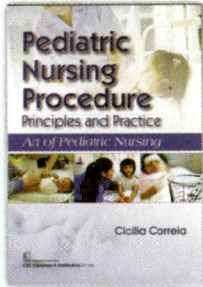

ISBN: 978-93-86310-74-3
Pages: 360   1/e, 2017

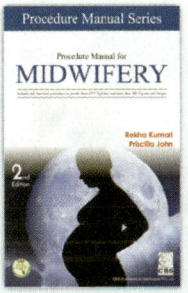

ISBN: 978-93-89261-94-3
Pages: 200   2/e, 2019

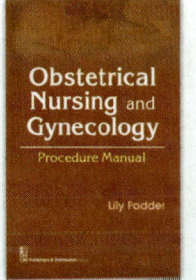

ISBN: 978-81-23925-81-3
Pages: 116   1/e, 2017

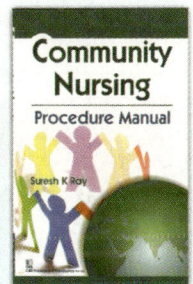

ISBN: 978-81-23929-35-4
Pages: 179   1/e, 2017

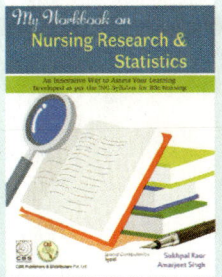

ISBN: 978-93-88108-75-1
Pages: 80   1/e, 2019

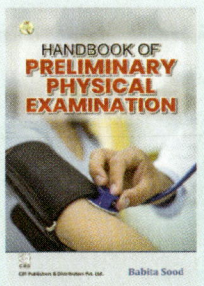

Releasing Soon

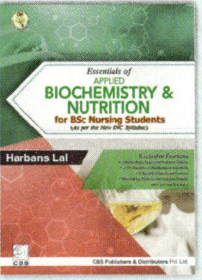

Releasing Soon

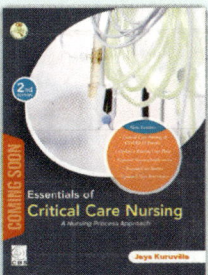

Releasing Soon

 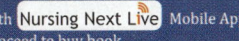
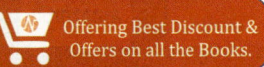

Common Title (BSc/GNM)

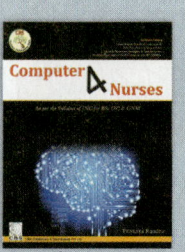

ISBN: 978-93-86310-48-4
Pages: 256   1/e, 2017

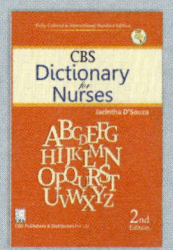

ISBN: 978-81-23927-16-9
Pages: 872   2/e, 2017

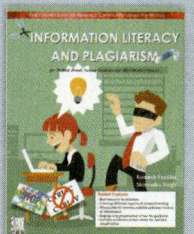

ISBN: 978-93-86827-13-5
Pages: 200   1/e, 2018

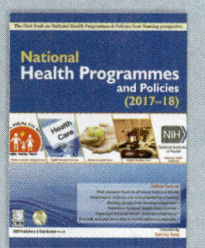

ISBN: 978-93-86310-43-9
Pages: 584   1/e, 2018

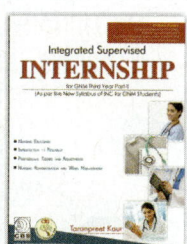

ISBN: 978-93-88108-89-8
Pages: 265   1/e, 2018

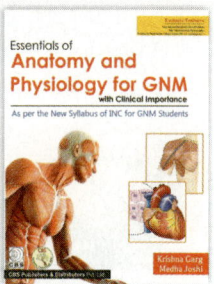

ISBN: 978-93-86827-11-1
Pages: 312   1/e, 2018

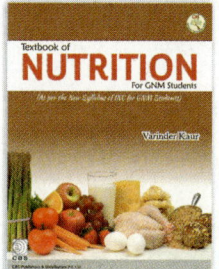

ISBN: 978-93-86827-10-4
Pages: 175   1/e, 2018

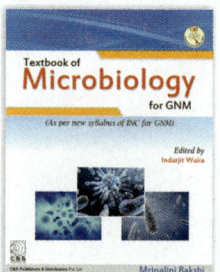

ISBN: 978-93-86827-23-4
Pages: 130   1/e, 2018

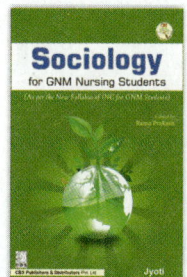

ISBN: 978-93-86827-26-5
Pages: 168   1/e, 2018

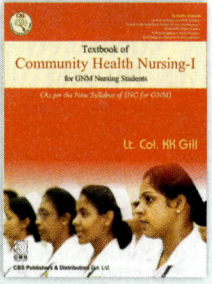

ISBN: 978-93-86827-17-3
Pages: 544   1/e, 2018

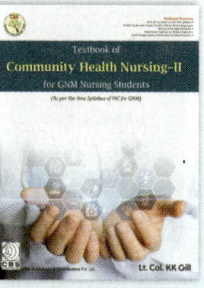

ISBN: 978-93-88178-57-0
Pages: 480   1/e, 2019

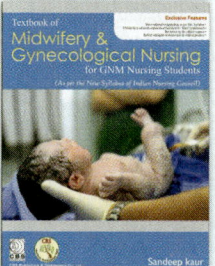

ISBN: 978-93-88108-83-6
Pages: 640   1/e, 2018

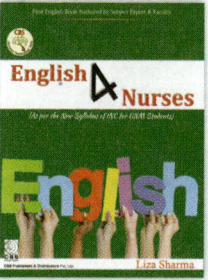

ISBN: 978-93-86827-09-8
Pages: 382   1/e, 2017

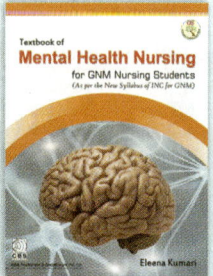

ISBN: 978-93-86827-48-7
Pages: 290   1/e, 2018

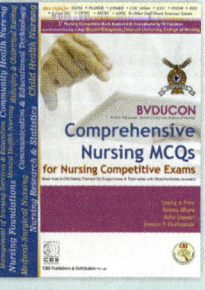

ISBN: 978-93-86310-33-0
Pages: 430   1/e, 2017

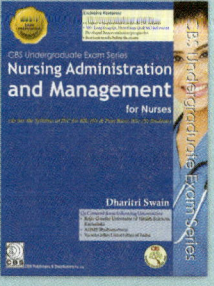

ISBN: 978-93-86827-42-5
Pages: 345   1/e, 2018

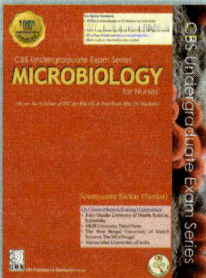

ISBN: 978-93-86310-49-1
Pages: 270   1/e, 2017

Nursing Undergraduate Exam Series

Buy online :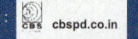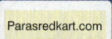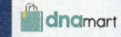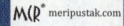

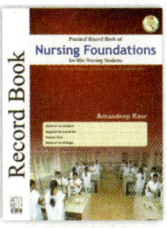

ISBN: 978-93-88108-96-6
Pages: 256   1/e, 2018-19

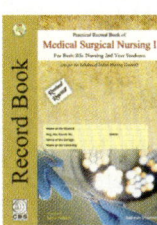

ISBN: 978-81-23928-00-5
Pages: 528   1/e, 2018-19

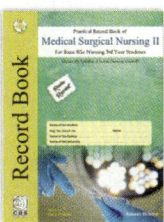

ISBN: 978-81-23928-01-2
Pages: 324   1/e, 2018-19

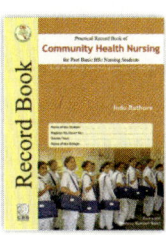

ISBN: 978-93-86827-06-7
Pages: 390   1/e, 2017

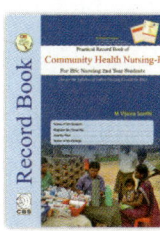

ISBN: 978-81-23926-84-1
Pages: 388   1/e, 2016

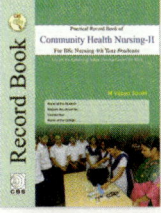

ISBN: 978-93-88108-77-5
Pages: 544   1/e, 2018-19

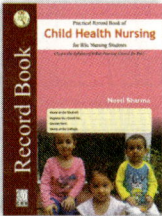

ISBN: 978-93-86827-05-0
Pages: 160   1/e, 2017

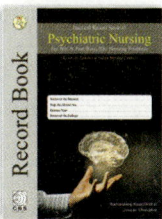

ISBN: 978-93-88108-80-5
Pages: 334   1/e, 2019

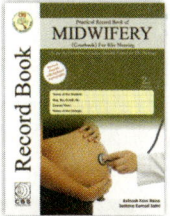

ISBN: 978-93-88178-65-5
Pages: 634   2/e (R/R), 2018-19

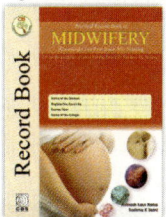

ISBN: 978-81-23927-07-7
Pages: 570   1/e, 2017

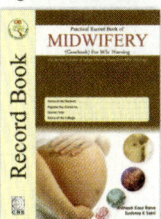

ISBN: 978-93-86217-97-4
Pages: 464   1/e, 2017

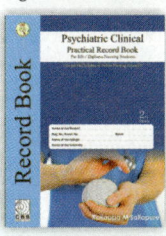

ISBN: 978-93-88108-81-2
Pages: 230   2/e, 2018-19

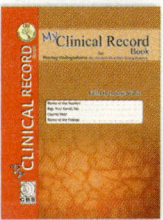

ISBN: 978-81-23927-04-6
Pages: 300   1/e, 2017-18

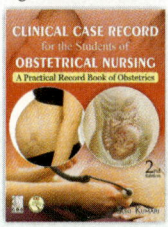

ISBN: 978-93-88178-51-8
Pages: 452   2/e, 2018

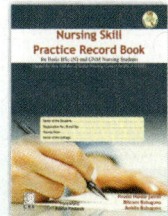

ISBN: 978-93-86827-38-8
Pages: 232   1/e, 2018-19

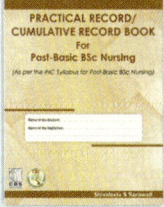

ISBN: 978-93-86827-02-9
Pages: 48   1/e, 2018

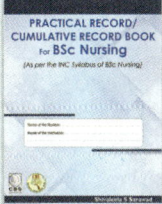

ISBN: 978-93-86827-01-2
Pages: 80   1/e, 2017

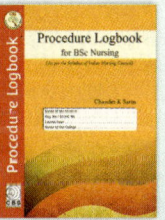

ISBN: 978-93-86310-46-0
Pages: 144   1/e, 2017

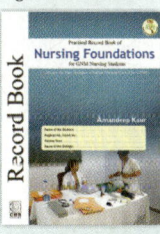

ISBN: 978-93-88178-50-1
Pages: 166   1/e, 2018-19

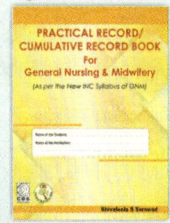

ISBN: 978-93-86827-03-6
Pages: 64   1/e, 2018

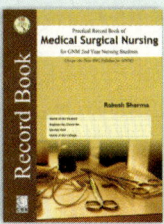

ISBN: 978-93-86827-04-3
Pages: 394   1/e, 2017

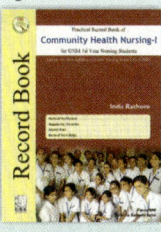

ISBN: 978-93-86827-07-4
Pages: 252   1/e, 2020

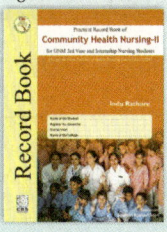

ISBN: 978-93-86827-30-2
Pages: 320   1/e, 2018-19

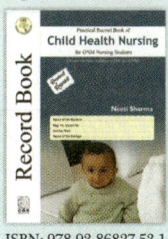

ISBN: 978-93-86827-53-1
Pages: 156   1/e, 2019

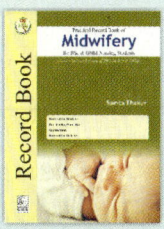

ISBN: 978-93-86827-33-3
Pages: 350   1/e, 2020

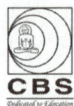

CBS PGMEE & Nursing Division

(A Unit of CBS Publishers & Distributors Pvt. Ltd.)

Sl. No. ☐☐☐☐☐☐☐   Date : D D M M Y Y Y Y

College Name: ☐☐☐☐☐☐☐☐☐☐☐☐☐☐☐☐☐☐☐☐☐☐☐☐☐☐☐☐☐

Contact Person Name: ☐☐☐☐☐☐☐☐☐☐☐☐☐☐☐☐☐☐☐☐☐☐☐☐☐☐☐

Email ID: ☐☐☐☐☐☐☐☐☐☐☐☐☐☐☐☐☐   Mob. No. ☐☐☐☐☐☐☐☐☐☐

Address: ☐☐☐☐☐☐☐☐☐☐☐☐☐☐☐☐☐☐☐☐☐☐☐☐☐☐☐☐☐

☐☐☐☐☐☐☐☐☐☐☐☐☐☐☐☐☐☐☐☐☐☐☐☐☐☐☐☐☐

City: ☐☐☐☐☐☐☐☐☐   State: ☐☐☐☐☐☐☐☐☐☐☐   Pin: ☐☐☐☐☐☐

Write in Capital Letters

Sl. No.	ISBN	Author	Title	Qty.	Discount
1	9789386827128	Indu Khurana	Textbook of Anatomy & Physiology for Nurses (2/e)		
2	9789388108942	Harindarjeet Goyal	Textbook of Nursing Foundations for BSc Nursing Students		
3	9788123927190	Harbans Lal	Essentials of Biochemistry for BSc Nursing Students		
4	9789389261950	Liza Sharma	English 4 Nurses for BSc(N) and BSc(N) Post Basic (2/e)		
5	9788123927114	Krishne Gowda	Essentials of Psychology for BSc Nursing Students		
6	9788123927138	Arora and Arora	Essentials of Microbiology for BSc Nursing Students		
7	9789388108829	Anju Dhir	Textbook of Microbiology for BSc & Post Basic Nursing Students		
8	9789389261929	Monika Sharma	Textbook of Nutrition for BSc Nursing Students (2/e)		
9	9789388108959	Sushma Pandey/ Mohd. Atif Muzammil	Principles & Procedures of Nursing Foundations (Volume I)		
10	9789389261875	Sushma Pandey/ Mohd. Atif Muzammil	Principles & Procedures of Nursing Foundations (Advanced Nursing Procedures) (Volume II)		
11	9789386310484	Priyanka Randhir	Computer 4 Nurses		
12	9788194523475	CP Thresyamma	Essentials of Basic Nursing Procedures (2/e)		
13	9789389261974	Sandhya Ghai	PGI Nine—Clinical Nursing Procedure (2/e), 2019		
14	9788123927169	Jacintha D'Souza	CBS Dictionary for Nurses		
15	9788123927046	Inderjit Walia	My Clinical Record Book for Nursing Undergraduates		
16	9789388178556	Sanju Sira	First Aid Manual for Nurses (2/e)		
17	9789389261882	Tarika Sharma/ Urvashi Sharma	ECG for Nurses		
18	9789386310460	Chander K Sarin	Procedure Logbook for BSc Nursing		
19	9789386827012	Shivaleela S Sarawad	Practical Record/Cumulative Record Book for BSc Nursing		
20	9789388108966	Amandeep Kaur	Practical Record Book of Nursing Foundation for BSc Nursing Students		
21	9789386217516	Krishne Gowda	Essentials of Sociology for BSc Nursing Students		
22	9789386217806	Joginder Pathania	Textbook of Pharmacology for BSc Nursing Students		
23	9788123927015	Shyamla D Manivannan	Textbook of Community Health Nursing-I		
24	9789388178587	L Gopichandran	Essentials of Communication & Education Technology for BSc Nursing (2/e)		
25	9788123928005	Rakesh Sharma	Medical Surgical Nursing Record Book—2nd Year		
26	9788123926841	M Vijaya Santhi	Practical Record Book of Community Health Nursing-I for BSc Nursing 2nd Year Students		
27	9789386827340	Ratna Prakash	Textbook of Nursing Education for BSc Nursing		
28	9789388178532	Yogesh Gulati, Rakesh Sharma	CBS Nursing Drug Guide 2020-21		
29	9789389261912	P Prakash	Textbook of Mental Health Nursing & Psychiatric Nursing for BSc Students		

Contd...

Sl. No.	ISBN	Author	Title	Qty.	Discount
30	9789388108812	Kallappa M Sollapure	Psychiatric Clinical Practical Record Book for BSc/Diploma Nursing Students		
31	9789386827050	Neeti Sharma	Practical Record Book of Child Health Nursing for BSc Nursing		
32	9788123928012	Rakesh Sharma	Medical Surgical Nursing Record Book-II-3rd Year		
33	9789388108805	Ramandeep Kaur Dhillon	Practical Record Book of Psychiatric Nursing for BSc and PBSc		
34	9789388178655	Avinash Rana	Practical Record Book of Midwifery (Casebook) for BSc Nursing (2/e)		
35	9789388108720	Meharban Singh/ Raman Kalia	Textbook of Pediatric Nursing for BSc Nursing Students		
36	9789388108867	Niyati Das	Procedure Manual for Pediatric Nursing		
37	9789388178518	Soni Kumari	Clinical Case Record for the Students of Obstetrical Nursing (A Practical Record Book of Obstetrics)—(2/e)		
38	9789389261943	Rekha Kumari	Procedure Manual for Midwifery		
39	9789389261899	Sukhpal Kaur, Amarjeet Singh	Nursing Research in 21st Century		
40	9789388108751	Sukhpal Kaur/ Amarjeet Singh	My Workbook on Nursing Research & Statistics		
41	9789388178617	T Sivabalan/G Vimala	Textbook of Nursing Research & Statistics for Undergraduates		
42	9789386217820	Reena J Wani	Textbook of Midwifery for Nurses		
43	9789386827227	Shyamla D Manivannan	Textbook of Community Health Nursing – II for BSc Nursing		
44	9789388178624	Beena MR/ Hari Krishna	Textbook of Nursing Management & Services for BSc Nursing		
45	9789388108775	M Vijaya Santhi	Practical Record Book of Community Health Nursing - II for BSc Nursing 4th Year Students		
46	9788123927077	Avinash Rana	Practical Record Book of Midwifery (for Post Basic BSc Nursing)		
47	9789386310439	Samta Soni	National Health Programmes and Policies (2017-18)		
48	9789388178600	Shweta Naik/ Hannah Roseline D	Procedure Manual for Obstetrics & Gynecological Nursing		
49	9789386827135	Ramesh Pandita/ Shivendra Singh	Information Literacy and Plagiarism		
50	9789386827029	Shivaleela S Sarawad	Practical Record/Cumulative Record Book for Post Basic BSc Nursing		
51	9789386217974	Avinash Kaur Rana/ Sushma Kumari Saini	Practical Record Book of Midwifery (Casebook) for MSc Nursing		
52	9789386827067	Indu Rathor	Practical Record Book of Community Health Nursing for Post BSc Nursing Students		
53	9789386310330	BVDUCON/Sneha A Pitre	BVDUCON Comprehensive Nursing MCQs		
54	9789386310446	Umesh Parashar	Smart Study Nursing Competition Manual		
55	9789386827388	Pratiti Haldar James	Nursing Skill Practical Record Book for Basic BSc(N) & GNM Nursing Students		
56	9789386310491	Soumyashree Sarkar	CBS Undergraduate Exam Series—Microbiology for Nurses		
57	9789386827425	Dharitri Swain	CBS Undergraduate Nursing Administration and Management for Nurses		
58	9789386827111	Krishna Garg/ Medha Josh	Essentials of Anatomy and Physiology for GNM		
59	9789386827104	Varinder Kaur	Textbook of Nutrition for GNM Students		
60	9789386827234	Mrinalini Bakshi	Textbook of Microbiology for GNM		
61	9789386827265	Jyoti	Sociology for GNM Nursing Students		
62	9789388178501	Amandeep Kaur	Practical Record Book of Nursing Foundation for GNM Nursing Students		
63	9789386827098	Liza Sharma	English 4 Nurses for GNM Students		
64	9789386827173	Lt Col. KK Gill	TB of Community Health Nursing-I for GNM		
65	9789386827036	Shivaleela S Sarawad	Practical Record/Cumulative Record Book for GNM Students		
66	9789386827074	Indu Rathor	Practical Record Book of Community Health Nursing-I for GNM 1st Year Nursing Students		
67	9789386827487	Eleena Kumari	Textbook of Mental Health Nursing for GNM Nursing Students		
68	9789388178563	Lt. Col KK Gill	Textbook of Environmental Hygiene for Nursing Students		
69	9789386827043	Rakesh Sharma	Practical Record Book of Medical Surgical Nursing for GNM 2nd Year Students		
70	9789386827302	Indu Rathor	Practical Record Book of Community Health Nurisng - II for GNM 3rd Year & Internship Nursing Students		
71	9789388178570	KK Gill	Textbook of Community Health Nursing-II		
72	9789388108836	Sandeep Kaur	Textbook of Midwifery & Gynecological Nursing GNM		
73	9789388108898	Taranpreet Kaur	Integrated Supervised Internship (for GNM-3rd Year)-Part-I		
74	9789386827333	Sarita Thakur	Practical Record Book of Midwifery for GNM Nursing Students		
75	9789386827531	Neeti Sharma	Practical Record Book of Child Health Nursing for GNM Nursing Students		
76	9789389261981	Muthuvenkatachalam	Target High-5th Premium Colored International Edition (5/e)		

Contd...

Sl. No.	ISBN	Author	Title	Qty.	Discount
77	9788194025658	Muthuvenkatachalam	Target High Hindi (2/e)		
78	9788194025603	Muthuvenkatachalam	Target CHO		
79	9788123929354	Suresh Ray	Community Nursing Procedure Manual		
80	9789386217875	Piyush Gupta	Essential Pediatric Nursing		
81	9789386310743	Cicilia Correia	Pediatric Nursing Procedure Principles and Practice Art of Pediatric Nursing		
82	9788123922140	Marie Elizabeth	Midwifery for Nurses		
83	9788123925813	Lily Poddar	Obstetrical Nursing & Gynaecology		
84	9788194523444	D R Arora, Brij Bala Arora	Essentials of Applied Microbiology for BSc Nursing (2/e), 2020-21		
85	TBA	Jacintha D'Souza	CBS Dictionary for Nurses English-Hinglish-Hindi (1/e), 2020-21		
86	TBA	Babita Sood	Handbook of Preliminary Physical Examination (1/e), 2020-21		
87	TBA	Harbans Lal	Essentials of Applied Biochemistry & Nutrition for BSc Nursing Student (1/e) 2020-21		
88	TBA	Jaya Kuruvilla	Essentials of Critical Care Nursing (2/e), 2020-21		